*my*Life Framework

A Model for a Successful Life based on the Yoga Principles

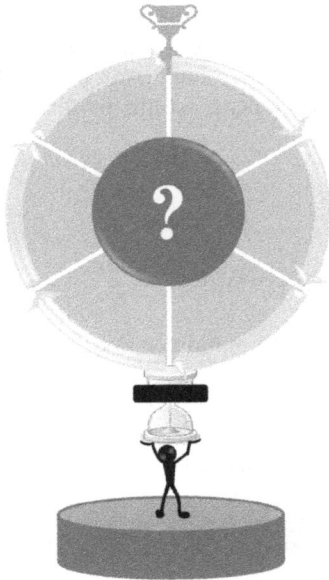

SUNIL SHEORAN

BharatPrem Publishing

ISBN: 0-9811921-0-6

ISBN/ EAN-13: 978-0-9811921-0-9

Register online for more information on this publication at
www.mylifeframework.com

Published in United States and Canada by BharatPrem Publishing

Printed in the United States of America

DEDICATION

This book is dedicated to my mother, Smt. Prem Kaur, and to all the mothers who play a very special role in our lives. I fall short of words for them – they are simply special.

CONTENTS

CHAPTER FIVE

Using the myLife Framework *131*

CHAPTER SIX

Concluding Thoughts *145*

LIST OF FIGURES

ABOUT THE BOOK

Contemporary popular culture promises us an unprecedented level of freedom to live our lives. It also presents too many continuously changing variables for us to make sense of life, let alone manage it effectively. There is too much noise around us to identify our appropriate role in the world and live a meaningful life. The new values of the global world, dominated by the West, are colliding with the established traditions of older cultures. No clear set of values seems to fill the vacuum for the "way of life" in today's dynamic world.

So how do I live a good life in these turbulent and noisy times?

When I tried answering this question, the journey was more complex and fascinating than I had originally imagined. This book is essentially the summary of this journey. Not all of us may have thought about this question directly, but subconsciously all of us make an effort to live a successful life. All of us want to improve our lives from today to tomorrow. However, be it internal improvement goals or the external measures of success, only a few of us achieve the personally set targets of a successful life.

One of the initial challenges on this journey of change is that most of us have an unclear, unstructured view of life. This ambiguity along with other factors results in a vague desire to improve oneself. Changing this vague desire into concrete steps to act upon isn't so easy though. This book provides a practical framework to structure all the aspects of our lives, which I call "the *my*Life Framework." The primary purpose of this book is to illustrate this framework, which I believe is very simple, comprehensive and flexible enough, to be adopted by all of us. By utilizing this framework, you can get a better sense of direction in life to harness the opportunities available in the modern world.

Example application of the *my*Life Framework in the book covers all the common aspects of human life, such as health, spirituality, relationships, money and desire fulfillment. The spiritual dimension presented in the book is based on the concepts of yoga. Yoga is a way of life and the science of spirituality that cuts through the seeming differences across religions. For people who are spiritual and religious, yoga provides the most logical way I have found to describe spiritual concepts. It also explains the commonalities and the reasons behind differences across religions. A proper understanding of yoga should help you not only appreciate other religions, but also improve your understanding of your own chosen path.

While many concepts in the book are derived from yoga, the framework itself is completely independent of yoga and spirituality. If you prefer, you can completely ignore the spiritual elements and still fully utilize the framework.

Life is supposed to be fun, but this book is not necessarily fun or a casual read. Indeed, it will force you to think at the deepest levels of your value system. With some analysis on the concepts in this book, I hope you will have a better understanding of human nature and an improved perspective on your own life. The content in this book is intended to serve as a one-time heavy dose of the principles of life, to help you do some quality thinking about it. This quality thinking will alleviate the need for ongoing unproductive thinking on the basics of life, and will help make life what it is supposed to be – fun!

There's great deal of philosophy and pop psychology all around us and I do not want to add more to it. The intent of the book is to stay focused at personal level so the text is short and direct, and contains only the necessary theoretical context. The book is not a philosophical exercise for conversational pleasures or to serve mind's lust of aimless analysis. For me, the goal was to develop a personal plan to ensure a better rest of my life. The idea of this analysis being valuable to others prompted me to document it in the form of this book.

Human beings are complex in many ways. The issues addressed in this book are equally complex and cover a very broad range. I don't claim to be a yoga guru or an expert in all these topics. This is my humble effort to share essential thoughts on life, as I understand them. I hope you benefit from my analyses and experiments. I also hope you will excuse any flaws in my analyses and only focus on the benefits you can extract from them.

The book offers many proven concepts and principles. Although essential guidance is provided to adopt these concepts, eventually you need to identify the ways to include these concepts in your own story of life. Just the way the taste of food is known only by eating it and not by reading the recipe, you will realize the value of the concepts discussed in this book, only by acting upon them. Reading books is just like getting the recipes; the value is limited to acquiring some information and some inspiration. I hope you will make the best use of the information presented in the book to improve your own life and the lives of others around you.

CHAPTER ONE

Introspection

How do I live a good life? What's the goal of life? How do I define a successful life for myself? How do I stay happy and healthy? How do I get love and respect from the people around me? And the list goes on...

Most of us think about these questions, or a variation of them, at least once in a while. These thoughts especially make their presence known when we are away from the hustle-bustle of everyday life, when we are true to ourselves and don't have the influence of the world pounding at us. Typically, before we can answer these questions to ourselves, or even contemplate them very deeply, we are back in our everyday lives, full of distractions.

Thoughts on life don't come in a structured way as the questions listed above. Our perspectives on life's big questions are subconsciously built by the environment we live in. Once we build these perspectives, it is pretty rare that we critique them with honest introspection.

The journey of life – The middle-class way

As a middle-class boy in India, brought up in an environment pretty conducive to personal growth, the viewpoint on life that I developed seemed straightforward. "Have fun as kids, get a good education, get a good job, raise a good family, and when we get old, our children take care of us." Perhaps I would also add "Be good, think about God, and help others as much as we can."

Obviously, this viewpoint is not as simple as it seems on the surface. As I grew, I saw many variations of this viewpoint and most of them made me uncomfortable. Life seemed not as pretty as I had subconsciously envisioned. I started realizing the challenges to accomplish the goals that supported my seemingly straightforward viewpoint of life.

Having fun as kids and getting an education was relatively simple in my case. But making money and noticing the shallowness of relationships were definitely big surprises to my subconscious childhood expectations. I found my goals to take some social responsibility and to explore spiritual truths were a distant consideration with the everyday struggles of personal life.

For everyone around me, the journey of life seemed to follow a similar pattern. As kids, most of them had pretty much the same experience and had a good time. As teenagers, most people had a lot of energy to do something positive. As their family protection decreased and the influence of the external environment increased, their lives started taking very different paths. In their 20s, everyone seemed to firm up their value systems and beliefs on life, albeit unknowingly. By their mid-30s, everyone seemed to struggle with pretty much the same things, dealing with the challenges of family life and efforts to make some *more* money. The general message from the older people was that the challenges of old age were worse than they had originally imagined.

This common journey of life was obviously very different from the childhood viewpoint on life, subconsciously built under our parents' protection.

Is this acceptable?

At some point during my teenage years, this thought stuck with me: "Is that it? Is life only about getting a job, raising a family, and being unhappy in old age? Is it acceptable to me?" Naturally, as we start thinking about anything philosophical, religion comes rushing into the analysis. As soon as we bring the spiritual or religious dimension, the questions take completely different shape. What's the purpose of human life? What is God? What is the origin of creation, and so on?

Being a student of science and being raised in a community where religion didn't drive our *way of life*, the concept of "God" didn't really make any sense to me at that time. Spiritual things being unprovable, I inadvertently started separating every analysis into two buckets – one spiritual and one regular (or logical). All the analysis of the "regular" world could be conducted by simple cause and effect logic, whereas the spiritual stuff went beyond any logic I could muster. The religious books suggested having "faith" in God, but didn't provide any real guidance on obtaining a proof of its existence. All these texts did was to tell me *how to live my life*, often in conflicting, confusing ways. So, although I didn't understand the spiritual stuff, separating the topic simplified the analysis around it.

In the same research phase, I read a few books on yoga and got some training in yoga therapy. Although I didn't have any health issues, yoga practice helped me feel more energetic, and I saw the positive results on my physical health right away. The evaluation of the results on my body and the more logical explanation of spiritual concepts convinced me to conduct further research in yoga philosophy. As I traveled to *ashrams* (hermitages) and spent time researching these topics, I saw no end to this research. This analysis definitely triggered some really good questions, some confusion and some answers.

One of the first important realizations I came to, was not to rely completely on my formal education for all the knowledge I needed. Instead, I came up with my own expectations of what I should get from my education. They included:

1. Education should provide me with professional skills to earn a living
2. Education should answer the big question, "How do I live a good life?"

After a while, I added a third one:
3. Education should make me a contributing member of the society and not a burden.

My formal education, I felt, was mostly superficial and essentially failed to fulfill these expectations. However, it did do a good job of helping me develop the professional skills I needed to earn a living. Developing these expectations from education, along with some other rules for myself, gave me confidence to have my own viewpoints and to question a lot of the established ways of thinking.

Introspection – What is the purpose?

I think all of us examine our thoughts to a certain extent; obviously, the quality of this self-examination varies drastically. Although I cannot recall all the initial incidents and sources that inspired me to get involved in self-analysis, the key motivating factors were claims made by authors in yoga literature. They all claimed the existence of forces beyond what our senses can capture and what modern science has discovered to date. They also suggested that every human being is capable of exploring these forces by following certain yogic methods.

Firmly keeping the spiritual aspects in a separate bucket, the logical questions I wanted to address were:

How do I define a successful life for myself? And how do I make sure that I live this personally defined successful life?

Although the lust of the mind to analyze stuff takes it everywhere, at the end of the day these were the two most basic questions for me. Somehow it always remained a priority for me to find the answers to these questions. I did try to figure out why it was important for me to find these answers, earlier rather than later. The first simple reason was that without these answers, poor or perfect, I felt that it was very difficult to manage day-to-day activities. I felt like I was losing control of life and becoming a puppet in the hands of popular culture, in which I could easily find quite a few flaws. I needed at least some *work in process* answers that could be used to pacify my mind. Also, I felt the danger of wasting the precious years of life on irrelevant things if I didn't have my own answers.

Influence of environment on our definition of successful life

From the very beginning of childhood we are continuously engaged in the world around us. We spend most of our time and mental energy juggling with the "external environment," as opposed to evaluating ourselves. There's no formal training in schools or at home on how to conduct introspection and build our definitions of a successful life. We are not really taught to have the independence of thought necessary to create our own definition of success. But without this independence, the world around us defines *how to live* and suggests accepting the established ways of thinking and living.

In Indian scriptures, the whole world or the *creation* operates on the basic principles of relativity and duality. Working on these principles, this *creation* called *"maya"*, ignorance or illusion, and is considered very tricky for all of us to overcome. An introduction to yoga philosophy in the spirituality section, explains this concept in more detail. The key point from this spiritual reference is that the environment we surround ourselves is of utmost importance, and is typically the primary driver of how we live our lives.

Acknowledging the strong influence of the external environment and striving for the independence of thought, I made a sincere effort to evaluate whatever happened around me. Additionally, I conducted research to understand the essence of human nature and some of our deep-rooted needs. The goal of all this introspection effort was to build a viewpoint on a successful life with as much independent and rational thought as possible. All this analysis occurred in a relatively unstructured way, as opposed to the thought process presented here.

What if, the popular culture defines success for us?

Power, fame and money! Traditionally, these three have been the symbols of a successful life and are true today as well. I think these are all right things to aim for, as they typically provide a good collection of experiences and their pursuit might help us discipline our lives, give us feelings of accomplishment, and hopefully improve our understanding of life itself. Inherently, there is nothing wrong with power, money and fame, but how we build the story of our life to include these external measures of success deserves some additional evaluation.

These external measures of success (e.g., power, fame and money) are manifested in different ways at different times in history. Let us look at some of the macro trends in the world today and see how they impact us on a personal level. Although there are quite a few positive elements in current popular (pop) culture, I'm focusing a bit more on its negative consequences for our personal lives in order to bring up some warnings as we think about our definition of success.

In the context of a definition of a successful life, I see **"globalization dominated by the Western world"** as the contemporary theme. Globalization goes way beyond integration of economies. It is essentially restructuring of the world at numerous levels. It is colliding with the established personal and family value systems, it is changing the social orders and the role of governments, and it is accelerating the consumption of the Earth's limited natural resources. Globalization is a reality of the future and we don't need to fight it or run away from it. In fact, we *have to* learn to absorb it in our lives. Although there are a lot of positive and negative consequences of globalization, what is its impact on our view of a successful life?

Improved information availability is one of the basic elements of today's global culture. During one of my recent travels, I was amazed to see how much information a small-town high school student in India had about America. With this global information comes a global comparison. Now for this high school student, the measure of success doesn't stop at his successful family members or neighbors, because his comparison is global! A lot of people want to be as rich as Warren Buffet or the Google founders and as famous as Tom Cruise or David Beckham. The point is, the culture of **global**

comparison is setting impossible and inappropriate standards of success for most of us, and an inability to reach our personally defined targets of success only brings frustration.

Another element of the West dominated globalization is **consumerism**. One of the key concepts in consumerism culture is "growth" (as opposed to development or progress). Popular consumerism culture suggests that we must consume at an accelerating pace to be considered valuable in the society. We must work hard; interact with the media and with people who expect us to spend our hard-earned money on consuming things. The natural outcome of this is to fall into debt so that the economy keeps moving, and we have to keep earning more money to pay for what we consumed with borrowed funds. People who run this show seem to have a relatively short-term view. Corporations focus on their quarterly performance and governments focus on their four- or five-year tenures. This commercial culture is hitting the limits of natural resources *very* fast, and is straining on our personal budgets.

One of the offshoots of too much commercialization is *instant gratification.* Just like fast food, the popular culture suggests expediting everything. The life cycle of a lot of things is decreasing with this belief. Job durations are shrinking, job locations are changing fast and relationships are becoming more transient. In this kind of popular culture, if our definition of success is impacted by mainstream media, we need to understand that most of the information we receive from the media is provided for commercial reasons.

Another warning from the popular culture is – **individualism**. It has been a cornerstone value in capitalism to drive competition and innovation. On the flip side, individualism works against building human bonds and drives us to be more self-centered. As the individualism-centric culture encourages personal freedom, the social pressures to sacrifice anything for the good of a broader community are pushed to the background. It is becoming more acceptable – in some cases, fashionable – to break any and every tradition in the name of personal freedom and to be called modern or contemporary. As humans, we are enjoying the personal freedom that comes with individualism. At the same time, we are social beings and are missing bonds with each other and with our established traditions, etc. As we define our own success, we owe a viewpoint to ourselves on *individualism*.

In essence, contemporary popular culture presents a lot of new opportunities, along with too many continuously changing variables for us to effectively manage our lives. There is too much noise around us to define a meaningful life with some certainty. The new values of the west-dominated global world are colliding with the established traditions of older cultures. In this fast-changing world, an established "way of life" in most countries no longer has a place. With all the noise, the established roles of people are being questioned all the time. There seems to be a significant confusion about our own *role* in these changing times as well. On the positive side, if we proactively take charge, the changes in the world also provide us a lot of freedom to define our place – our "role" in the world.

What is the essence of human nature?

Yes, the external environment mentioned above is very powerful and keeps prescribing the way of life for most of us. So many of us are angry, frustrated and depressed because we cannot accomplish our impossible dreams. Because of the high-spending culture, many of us are in financial debt. Due to the mainstream media and individualism, sex-focused male/female relationship is getting viewed as the primary human relationship. And the list of challenges continues...

With some of these thoughts, I obviously questioned popular culture to define the way of life for me.

To define a *way of life* for me, I wanted to understand some of the key characteristics and deeper needs we have as human beings. Numerous generations have lived life before us and I wanted to get some timeless lessons from their life experiences. If I could understand the essentials of human nature, perhaps I could also make better sense of the world around me. I conducted some research in biology, anthropology and history in pursuit of this knowledge about the essence of human nature. For me, the focus moved very quickly to yoga philosophy, which seemed to address the issues of life at a much more foundational level.

Since yoga is primarily a spiritual field, I had to derive themes for human psychology, biology, social aspects, and so on. Based on yoga theory, human behavior can be described with the following logic:

Our five sense instruments gather data from the world around us. The data from these instruments is analyzed by the sense centers in our brain. These five sense centers of sight, touch, hearing, smell and taste are well recognized. The analysis ability inside us has two dimensions – thinking and feeling. Each of these two dimensions has two sides – positive and negative (good and bad). In yoga, the good and bad are described based on how our thoughts or feelings work against or in support of reaching spiritual goals. For our purposes, let's ignore the spiritual aspect for now and address the good side or bad side in terms of their effect on any desired goal. All this analysis inside us results in three things:

1. Identification of certain goals that we want to achieve,
2. A certain level of will power to accomplish the identified goals, and

3. Manifestation of our ego as our attachments. The term ego here is not the same as pride. In yoga, it is essentially how we identify ourselves; it is what we call "me" and "mine." This is sort of our answer to the question, "Who am I?" knowingly or unknowingly. Our most basic attachment is considered to be with our own body.

A more detailed explanation of yoga theory is presented later in the book, but here I want to share two specific outcomes from yoga that relate to the essence of human nature. I know I'm digressing from the definition of a successful life and introspection to explain these yoga concepts but I believe the awareness of these two outcomes will help you better absorb some of the concepts discussed later in the book. The two outcomes I observed are:

1. A three-dimensional framework to evaluate ourselves, other individuals and broader communities
2. Two universal laws that drive all the results or outcomes in our lives

Criteria to evaluate ourselves and the world around us

As we evaluate people (sometime ourselves), communities and circumstances around us all the time, I wanted to have a standard way to analyze the rationale behind things. From my understanding of yoga theory, I've found the three dimensions of *strength*, *wisdom* and *ego* to be pretty helpful in this regard which correspond to the three results of the subconscious analysis mentioned above – identification of goals, a level of will power and manifestation of our ego. These three internal dimensions of *strength*, *wisdom* and *ego* interact with each other to drive our everyday behavior as we interact with our external environment.

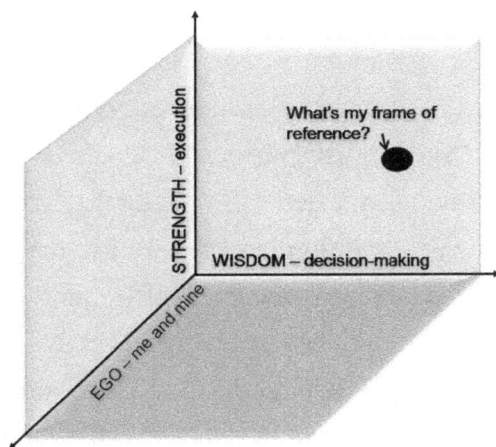

Figure 1: Three dimensions to evaluate individuals and societies

Wisdom is our ability to make right decisions. It is about what is the right thing to do? Clarity of mind, calmness and concentration directly impact our ability to make the right decisions. Traits like a desire to learn, being rational, and open-mindedness align with wisdom. On the flip side, there are numerous reasons to make inappropriate decisions, the most common of which are ignorance, fear and bias. Typically, biases originate from tradition, religion, value systems, habits and attachment to *me* and *mine* (ego). Biases start anywhere and everywhere, and they end at the ego and the body. At the community level, typically the older the culture is, the more traditions it has, the higher the probability of biases. The key takeaway here is that biases run deep inside us as individuals and collectively as a society. We need to consider our own biases and the biases of the object of our observation as we make decisions in life.

Strength serves as a measure of independence and our ability to execute and accomplish our desired goals. Fearlessness is the main virtue suggested in yoga that supports this dimension. There is a higher probability that a stronger person would be able to become self-reliant more easily. Practically, strength may not be always directly proportionate with the results people achieve in life. There are elements to consider, such as where people start and what kind of support structure they can leverage to accomplish desired goals. The *hierarchy of needs* concept can be used on this dimension to evaluate the independence of an individual or a society. The concept, credited to Abraham Maslow, suggests that there is an inherent order in the human needs to be fulfilled. Broadly, two categories can be used to build a quick viewpoint. The first category is the group whose *basic needs* of life are met, while the second category is the one struggling to meet their basic needs. The definition of basic needs can definitely be argued, of course. In today's culture, basic needs would include physical needs and security for health, family, employment, etc. Eventually, they need to be defined by the person or society under evaluation.

Ego defines how an individual or a society views its relationship with everything around it. As humans, we are connected with or attached to the people and everything else around us in numerous ways. Whatever we connect with, we always try to defend it. The objects of attachment become part of our identity. This attachment could be with people, material objects, ideas, traditions or anything else. The strength of the attachment is directly tied to the strength of obsession with the object of attachment. For example, this obsession could very well be with *success* or *defending our identity*, in whatever way we define it. When we are attached to something, it is not easy to discriminate between the observer and the object of observation and this attachment could very well blind the dimensions of wisdom and strength.

An understanding of connectedness provides a good insight into the intent of people's objectives and behaviors.

As an example at the individual level, I would want to be as unbiased as possible on the wisdom axis in order to make the right decisions in life. Being wise or rational would require me to genuinely question my own traditions and preconceived notions. On the strength dimension, I'd obviously want to focus on improving my ability to execute and make an effort to fulfill basic needs as soon as possible to become more independent. As desires are never ending, I have to make up my mind about the scope of my basic needs. On the "me and mine" (ego) dimension, I would want to have deep relationships with family and a few others, while leaving them sufficient personal independence. With this example of my personal *frame of reference*, I can start evaluating other individuals in relation to where I stand.

As an example evaluation of broad societies, let us do a quick comparison of India and America. We can rank India pretty high on tradition and biases due to its old culture and heritage, pretty high on *me* and *mine* due to extended family culture, and relatively low on independence. This is justifiable, as a significant portion its billion plus population cannot get enough opportunities to explore their potential and become independent in a hierarchical society. In comparison, America can be very quickly tested with the same three dimensions. It would also rate pretty high in tradition, but much less than India, relatively low on ego or connectedness because individualism is a primary value of the society; and it would rank very high on meeting the basic needs of its citizens with huge amounts of available resources.

Although the analysis of a community or society is different from that of an individual, I've been able to find pretty quickly a nuance of the three basic dimensions of strength, wisdom and ego to conduct appropriate analysis. Without a framework, our analysis is solely dependent upon our expertise in every situation under evaluation. This framework has helped me conduct some in-depth analyses and also has aided me in quickly making up my mind on something specific in fast-paced day-to-day life.

Two universal laws

Since we constantly work to fulfill our desires, one after another, fulfillment of desires is one of the ways to look at life. I've observed two laws from yoga theory that drive accomplishment of results in order to fulfill our desires. These laws are universally applicable to all human beings and align with the logic of human behavior discussed earlier.

These are: the *law of free-will* and the *law of cause and effect*. A regular reminder about and practice of these two laws can provide a better control of life by helping us to identify and accomplish the right goals.

1. *The Law of Free-Will:* The law says, "We always have freedom to make decisions." This law suggests that a person must take complete control of and accountability for life by freely making the right decisions. A practitioner of this law can never be a pessimist. Because we need to make success happen in our thoughts before it actually materializes, being an optimist or proactively taking charge is a fundamental requirement of a successful life. This law does not suggest that external circumstances are always going to be supportive of our goals. It is important to differentiate between pressures of the external environment and the concept of independence in making choices. Spiritually speaking, humans are made in the image of God, and we are capable of doing everything that God is capable of doing. It is *maya,* or illusion, that clouds our divinity and suggests that we are weak or incapable of accomplishing certain things.

    This law drives the first step in accomplishing any results based on the logic of human behavior mentioned previously in this chapter. Forgetting or not practicing this law is one of the primary reasons we don't achieve the results we desire. It is lack of our awareness, understanding, and/or getting convinced of our inability to achieve results that stops us from practicing this law.

Whatever external circumstances may exist, a practitioner of this law makes conscious, proactive decisions based on the desired outcome.

2. *The Law of Cause and Effect:* The law says, "If there's an action, there's always a corresponding result." This law is applicable to everything in nature, not just our lives. As we are always working to get some desired result, this law guides us to create the *cause* of that desired result. Consciously using this law simplifies life drastically by taking the focus away from unproductive thinking and putting it on the right activity to produce the results we want. This is the second step in accomplishing any results based on the logic of human behavior.

An important derivation of this law is the concept of habit in which repeated actions and outcomes become *the habit* of a person. These habits could be either positive or negative, depending upon whether they help us go towards our desired goals. In Hindu scriptures, this law suggests that after we go through the consequences of our actions, an impression is still left, which is called *sanskaar*.

In essence, our thoughts lead to actions which produce results. After we experience the results or consequences of our actions, we are still left with our habits and *sanskaar*. The scriptures suggest that we start our next life exactly with what we bring from previous life as habits or *sanskaar*.

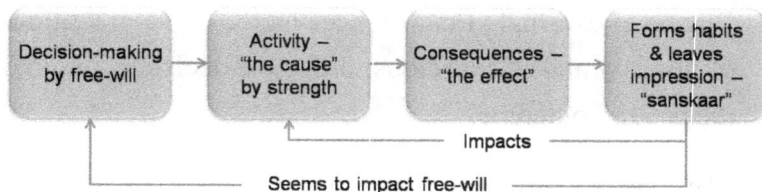

Figure 2: Two universal laws

Take charge to define "my successful life" – A suggested viewpoint

Our thoughts may wander around philosophy and the world for some time but, sooner or later, introspection always brings the focus back to the self. So how does all this thinking apply to me? If I believe in the cause and effect law, what "effects" do I want and what "causes" do I need to work on? If I use three-dimensional analysis, where do I stand now and where do I want to be? For the strength dimension, I need to evaluate my upbringing, my parents and family tree to identify and leverage my strengths and watch out for weaknesses. For the wisdom dimension, I need to stay alert and keep learning my whole life! For the ego dimension, I need to be careful about what I call me and mine, and be aware of how much of it is personal, how much is related to the external world, and how much is spiritual. If I believe in the *law of free will*, I have decisions to make, and if I'm made in the image of God, I'm capable of doing anything and everything!

Starting with the fulfillment of desires viewpoint, I built a rough list of goals to accomplish in life. With some logical reasoning and by combining spiritual thoughts of controlling my desires, I prioritized the list of things to happen in my life. This prioritization exercise, and cutting out some items made me think that it's a state of mind I'm going after. Furthermore, it is simply my belief that the desired state of mind can be achieved via the accomplishment of my goals. This state of mind is sometimes excitement, sometime calmness, sometimes satisfaction and sometimes happiness.

It was an "aha" moment for me to get the focus away from the accomplishment of goals to a state of mind. I thought, "That's it! The goal of life is having a desired state of mind, a desired feeling, all the time." Let me call this desired state a happiness that never dies. So, if I'm happy all the time that would be a successful life.

However, it is too vague and philosophical to zero in on a feeling of happiness or satisfaction. Obviously, we still need to and want to *do* things in life. For all the things in my list, I still had to create all the *causes* for the desired *effects* to happen. Later on, I read somewhere that everything in nature is in motion. Activity is a natural law and we simply can't be inactive. As Einstein said, "Life is like riding a bicycle. To keep your balance, you must keep moving."

With this kind of thought process, my introspection came down to two conclusions. One was that the goal of life is *"ongoing happiness that never dies"*, and two was the need to *"balance efforts proactively"* to accomplish our external goals. I also concluded that the *ongoing happiness* is not possible by avoiding all pains and accumulating more and more pleasurable events. Along with other things, it is feasible only with a sincere effort focused on the continuous goal of *even-mindedness.*

After separating a successful life into internal states of mind and specific goals in the external world, everything looked simpler. Before I reached these two very simple conclusions, figuring out the answer for "how do I live a good life?" felt like an insurmountable challenge.

With these two conclusions and everything I had analyzed to this point, putting together the *"my*Life Framework" was relatively simple. However, the path traveled to reach these conclusions was neither short nor without hiccups.

CHAPTER TWO

The myLife Framework

With the concepts of *happiness* and *balance*, the next logical step for me was to structure my ideas for execution. It was a very uncomfortable feeling to keep thinking about the basic stuff, without much progress in execution. I was keen to end all this heavy-duty thinking and get to the execution part with a *clearly identified direction* in my life. This led to the need for a framework.

Expectations from the *my*Life Framework

The goal of any framework is to structure things. The framework would help me organize thoughts on life in a simple and usable way. This *my*Life Framework should be the anchor to bring back the constantly wandering, inconsequential thoughts. Human beings are a *single, inseparable entity*, with different physical, mental, emotional, and spiritual aspects and this framework should cover *all* these aspects of life. When I'm old, I should be able to say to myself that I have lived a good life and this framework was vital to it. To me, the concern of not living a good life was quite a serious one. The big challenge was to summarize ALL my thinking in a concise and meaningful way and the constantly changing thoughts only made this challenge more difficult.

The law of cause and effect suggests that I'm supposed to focus on execution, but some high-level directional thinking is still needed before getting to execution. The framework should work as the strategy of my life, so it should capture the definition of my successful life. The framework should also work as an operating model for my life and help me make tactical plans for execution. With upfront planning taken care of, the execution should be smoother and save me precious time while building good habits. Since I believed we are what our habits are, the framework should help me build good habits for my spiritual quest. Along with the internal aspects of satisfaction and happiness, the framework should help me become successful in the material world. The framework had no small job to do!

The *my*Life Framework overview

With these lofty expectations from the "*my*Life Framework", I started thinking about all the variables to be included in the framework and how to structure them in a simple, usable format. Here's the graphic and elements of the *my*Life Framework that I came up with:

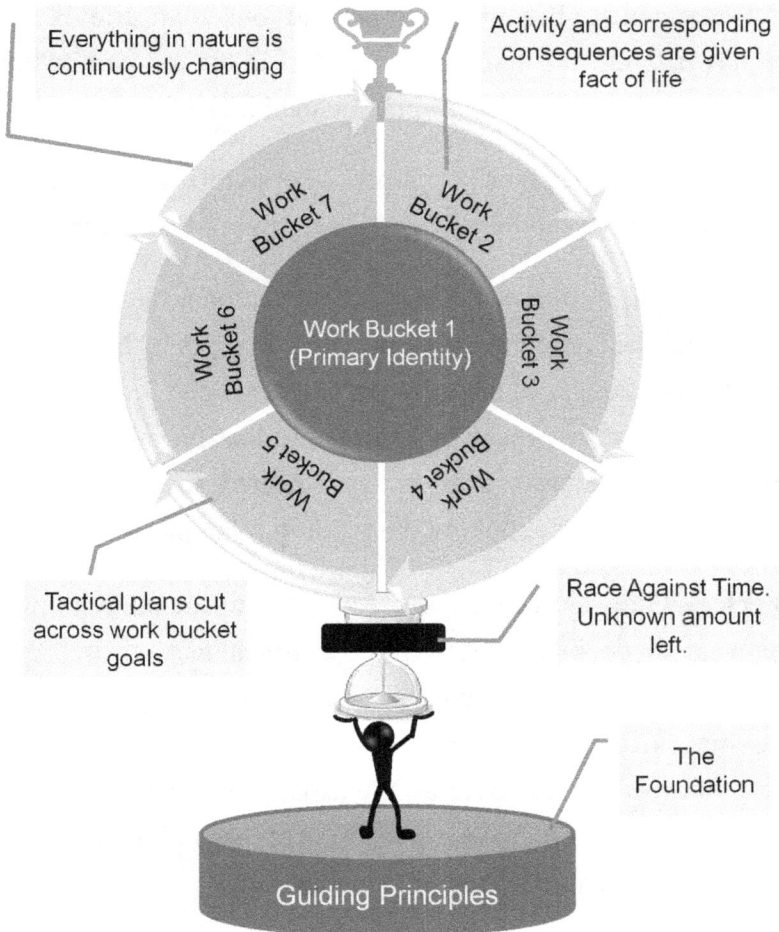

Everything in nature is continuously changing

Activity and corresponding consequences are given fact of life

Work Bucket 7

Work Bucket 2

Work Bucket 6

Work Bucket 1 (Primary Identity)

Work Bucket 3

Work Bucket 5

Work Bucket 4

Tactical plans cut across work bucket goals

Race Against Time. Unknown amount left.

The Foundation

Guiding Principles

Figure 3: The *my*Life Framework

Time is the most common denominator in life, as death is a certainty for all of us. We have finite time available to us, and the clock is continuously ticking. The hourglass held up by the human figure illustrates the limited amount of time available, which is unknown. Yes, there is an average human life expectancy, but the time left in our own life is an unknown. Thus, the amount of sand left in the top part of the hourglass is hidden in the graphic by the black bar

Although I'm not going to harp on the significance of time, the value of time should be considered of utmost importance.

The Guiding Principles are a few foundational thoughts that drive our behavior throughout life. Everyone has these guiding principles, knowingly or unknowingly. Ideally, we need to make a proactive effort to identify our guiding principles. (The next chapter is dedicated to providing a viewpoint and an example of the guiding principles.)

Work Buckets are needed to organize all of the many things we want to do in life. Activity is a given fact of life. We simply cannot be inactive, so we need to organize our activities in certain buckets or categories. Collectively, the work buckets should cover all the aspects of our life without any overlap. Although these work buckets are interdependent, any overlap is a sign of ambiguous thinking.

Goals are specific targets to achieve within each work bucket. The overall goals of life are a collection of specific goals within work buckets.

Tactical Plans are the high-level plans of work to achieve the goals within and across the work buckets. As different goals compete for our time and effort, the interdependency of the work buckets need to be considered. The basic elements of a tactical plan are a list of tasks to be executed, amount of time it takes and timing for tasks, and their interdependencies. All of the high-level tactical plans eventually roll into a single execution plan and a personalized daily routine.

Results are the rewards or negative consequences of our actions. The trophy in the graphic represents the results of our efforts across all the work buckets. Spiritually speaking, results are the fruits of all our *karma* or action, and an impression of our *karma* is carried to the next life. With or without spiritual consideration, the results are the consequences of our work. These consequences also leave a memory of experience and firm up our habits that impact our future behavior.

Continuous Motion or continuous change in life is illustrated by the circular arrows around the work buckets. In a spiritual context, this also highlights our next lives and *yugas*, a concept explained in more detail later in the book.

All of us do everything mentioned in this framework, mostly subconsciously. However, we need to be more conscious about the dynamics of this framework within our own lives, with the goal to improve it. Without taking charge of our lives in this way, we are nothing more than puppets in the hands of our old habits and our environment.

An example application of the *my*Life Framework is demonstrated in Figure 4 to provide additional clarification of the core concepts. This application is generic enough for a broad range of people to get started with the *my*Life Framework. The next two chapters illustrate the guiding principles and the work buckets components of the framework.

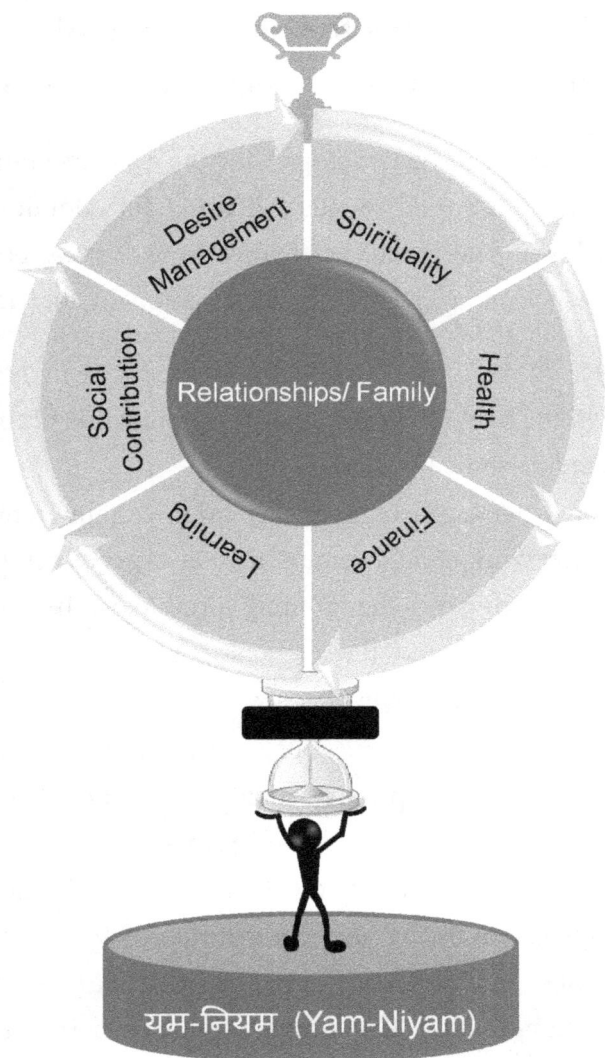

Figure 4: The *my*Life Framework – Example application

Guidelines for adoption and personalization of the *my*Life Framework

Some rules need to be developed for the *my*Life Framework to make the conceptual foundation ready for adoption at the personal level. The guidelines below are a starting point and provide a common ground for explanation in the next two chapters.

- The living and breathing *my*Life Framework needs to be updated periodically

- Although we can change it any time, certain elements of the framework should remain firm at every given point of time. Specifically, the guiding principles, list of work buckets, goals, and the tactical plans to achieve them should be unambiguous.

- There's only one work bucket (the center piece) that corresponds to the primary identity or *central theme* of a person's life. The concept of primary identity helps a person define his or her role in life or place in the world. This helps alleviate the competition between multiple identities and makes work prioritization easier. In challenging times, this primary identity helps decision-making become easier due to our proactively identified *role* and importance of things in life. In spirituality, the concept of *role* is known as one's *dharm* or *dharma* or the purpose of life. In the example application above, relationships/ family is the primary identity, but you can put whatever you feel is your primary identity in the center spot.

- Just like other work categories, the primary identity work bucket may also change. Practically the likelihood of changing might be less, but yoga theory suggests that it will change. The concept is that we identify ourselves with body or mind, and both of them are constantly changing.

- The concept of balance suggests that we consciously decide the amount of time and mental energy for each work bucket. It does not imply spending equal of effort in each work bucket.

- Timing is important, as is the balance of work buckets throughout life. For example, sick people would make an extra effort to become healthy, whereas financially poor people would try to earn more money, in order to become financially independent.

- As we mature or progress in our life, the amount of effort we put into specific work buckets keep changing. Everyone has a different understanding of the word *progress*. To me, *progress* has been part of life's viewpoint along with the concepts of *happiness* and *balance*. As we *progress in life*, we must be able to *spend more time and mental energy into higher level of activities, more freely*. Spiritually, meditation is the highest form of activity, so the range of activities includes becoming materially self-reliant to meditating. You need to have your own definition of progress while utilizing the *my*Life Framework.

- To qualify as a work bucket, we need to spend a minimum amount of work effort on that area. For example, if *health* is a work bucket and we do nothing to take care of it, it doesn't qualify as a work bucket.

- To get results, the concept of mental energy needs to be considered along with the investment of time. I'm using the generic term *mental energy* to include *any* and *every* thinking work we do. As a small example, during the process of writing this book, once it took me a couple of months to finish a single paragraph because of my constant travel and work pressure during that time. Although I had enough time to write the content, my mental energy was spent somewhere else during that period, to produce even a paragraph.

- As humans are a single, inseparable entity, the work buckets are interdependent. The tactical plans for work need to consider this interdependency of the work buckets to drive execution.

- The goals within work buckets and corresponding tactical plans are more dynamic than the guiding principles and work bucket definitions, which should remain relatively stable. Once our guiding principles and work buckets are well established, I don't see them changing every few months or even every year. They do need to be reviewed periodically – once a year or so. The goals and tactical plans are obviously more dynamic and need a varying timeline review, such as monthly, quarterly, every six month etc.

- For execution, the focus needs to be on a single, prioritized plan of work. The quality of this "one" execution plan is a direct result of the upfront effort put into personalizing the framework, with honest introspection and diligence in tactical planning.

The abovementioned rules for adoption of the *my*Life Framework should not be considered limiting or comprehensive for each one of us. One should build upon these guidelines to personalize the framework for his or her own use.

In the absence of this framework, there is a risk of focusing on narrow goals and ignoring the important aspects of life. Additionally, without the holistic view of life enabled by a well-defined framework; the unplanned goals keep changing all the time.

My experience suggests that even without the specific details on its elements, only a personalized skeleton of this framework provides a much clearer direction in life. Ambiguities begin to vanish, and one starts spending time on more relevant activities. With some details on guiding principles and work buckets, the framework is ready for execution.

CHAPTER THREE

The Guiding Principles –
An Example

Even before I had the first thought on the *my*Life Framework, I felt the need for some foundational principles to guide my life. Without some basic principles I had to always wonder about the basis of my decision-making. Having a perfect or close-to-perfect list of personal principles, a few foundational thoughts actively in mind seemed to make a lot of sense. For most of us, these principles are unplanned and are natural outcomes of our life experiences. The guiding principles acquired subconsciously cannot ever be basic enough or broad enough and will be incomplete to cover every aspect of our lives. As shown in Figure 5, the subconsciously acquired random "rules" to live by would be too many, and would be imperfect to serve as building blocks of life.

So I decided to identify my guiding principles proactively, without which I simply could not have a meaningful viewpoint on life itself.

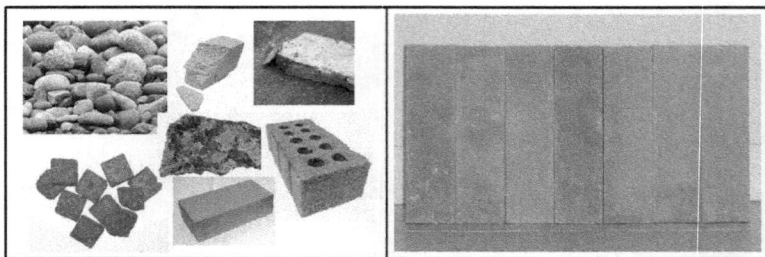

Figure 5: Guiding principles – Proactively identified vs. subconsciously acquired

How do we know our guiding principles are the right ones?

With some introspection, I started identifying my key guiding principles by making a list of some personal traits, favorite quotations and stories, and my own rules to live by. After building the initial list, the next logical step was to ensure the quality of the list. In the absence of a criterion, making a perfect list of guiding principles seemed impossible. I cross-checked my guiding principles against a list of traits I built around socially accepted norms of greatness. I compared my personalized list of traits against the lists in some business leadership and political leadership books. This exercise suggested that personal traits or guiding principles can be categorized – for example, strength and confidence could go into one category, and truth and rationality into another. The categories brought down the number of principles and improved the practical usage of these principles.

With some clarity and some confusion, none of these exercises seemed to make my list of guiding principles perfect or near perfect. I think human beings are pretty complex and we all build *our story of life* a bit differently. It is very difficult to summarize this complexity and its continuous interaction with external factors into a few principles. A strong desire to explore spiritual truths made my case even more complex. The big "aha" moment finally came when I compared *yam* and *niyam* of yoga with my list of guiding principles.

Yam and *niyam* are the first and second steps in the eight-step path of *rajyog* or *raja yoga*. This is the value system, the moral training to ensure progress on the spiritual journey. *Yam* is a set of five self-restraint principles intended to keep a practitioner focused on the path of spiritual development. *Niyam* is a set of five precepts, the directives that a spiritual aspirant practices regularly. These *yam-niyam* principles are the foundation of all the religions in Hinduism. As a clarification, Hinduism is a collection of many religions, which are different paths to spiritual evolution.

The *yam-niyam* principles are also claimed to be the basis of ALL the world religions. This made me think that the *yam-niyam* should be a complete and perfect set of guiding principles, and if not, then I could make them complete for me by personalizing them. Although the *yam-niyam* principles were originally developed for spiritual growth, I evaluated principles' effectiveness in everyday life. Nine out of the 10 *yam-niyam* principles convinced me of their depth and practicality in improving life. The last one, *dedication to God*, is a purely spiritual principle that intrigued me for quite some time.

As an experiment, I tested everyone I knew on the scale of *yam-niyam* principles, including myself. I noticed that the quality of a person's life and the *yam-niyam* principles tended to be in direct proportion. Knowingly or unknowingly, the lives of the happier people were better aligned with these principles. Considering humans as a single, inseparable entity, the *yam-niyam* principles covered all aspects of life – physical, mental, emotional, and spiritual. Some additional analysis convinced me that *yam-niyam* principles are complete for me. I needed some additional thoughts around the basic *yam-niyam* descriptions to make them more meaningful for me. All the previous analysis on guiding principles made this exercise relatively quick.

I invite you to test these *yam-niyam* guiding principles as complete and as the common, basic value system across all the religions. To conduct this test, one needs to have at least some spiritual bent of mind. Also, one needs to consider the possibility that other religions are also viable options, along with their own, to reach some common spiritual destination.

In the yoga context, I want to highlight the concept of *dharna*, the one-pointedness, the concentration. Any kind of spiritual practice should lead to a high level of concentration before providing any significant spiritual experience. In the spiritual journey, all the steps in *rajyog* prior to *dharna* (see the section on Spirituality for the eight steps in *rajyog*), including *yam-niyam*, can be viewed as enablers of *dharna* – the concentration.

An introduction to spirituality presented in the next chapter provides additional context on these principles. As *yam-niyam* principles are originally a spiritual value system, you might want to review these principles after reading the spirituality section.

Putting aside the spiritual aspect for now, *concentration* and *clarity of mind* are important for everything we do in life. This peaceful mind is also the prerequisite for the goal of life – that is, happiness. So these principles are relevant even if we don't consider anything spiritual. For the purpose of the *my*Life Framework, the *yam-niyam* principles are an example of the guiding principles component.

The yoga literature does have some variation in describing *yam-niyam* principles, particularly around the breadth of scope and around the depth of each principle. All the sources I investigated agree on the central theme though.

Overview of example guiding principles

Here's a brief definition of each of the *yam-niyam* principles, along with some additional thoughts

Yam, the self-restraint principles, include *satya* (truthfulness), *ahinsa* (non-violence), *asteya* (non-stealing), *aparigrah* (non-accumulation) and *brahamcharya* (sense control).

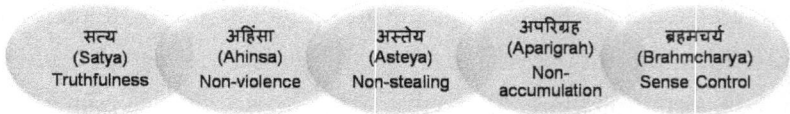

| सत्य (Satya) Truthfulness | अहिंसा (Ahinsa) Non-violence | अस्तेय (Asteya) Non-stealing | अपरिग्रह (Aparigrah) Non-accumulation | ब्रह्मचर्य (Brahmcharya) Sense Control |

Figure 6: *Yam* – The self-restraint principles

1. *Satya* **(truthfulness):** For everything the senses observe, analysis without any bias and an exact communication back to the world is called *satya*.

Being truthful requires curbing our selfishly biased intentions. The yoga literature suggests combining it with the welfare of everyone. If a truth will hurt others, staying quiet and away from those circumstances is recommended. Being truthful requires a lot of strength, fearlessness, and the ability to bear consequences. The reward includes improved will power, fearlessness, and significant reduction in the number of variables one has to deal with. This simplification directly feeds into being peaceful, which is a prerequisite of happiness and is an enabler of improved concentration.

2. *Ahinsa* **(non-violence):** Non-injury to others by thoughts, words or deeds is called *ahinsa*.

The key thought here is not having a *desire* to hurt anyone. The practice of *ahinsa* curbs jealousy towards people around us. One automatically becomes a well-wisher of everyone, which is the foundation of all good relationships. Depending upon circumstances, the literal practice of *ahinsa* may not be practical, so focusing on *desire not to hurt anyone* is of higher significance. In fact, every religion preaches non-violence and all of them have exceptions when violence is justified. History is full of bloodshed due to religions using these exceptions to non-violence.

3. *Asteya* **(non-stealing):** Non-stealing by thoughts or deeds is called *asteya*.

Again, the primary focus is on taming the *desire* to acquire the material assets owned by someone else. This translates into control of greed and being satisfied with the fruits of one's own hard work. The yoga literature suggests that our narrowness of mind is responsible for making us conceal and steal. A narrow mind constrains our connectedness to only the objects of our possession. If we don't understand ourselves as an integral part of nature, our ability to enjoy the wealth of the world becomes limited.

4. *Aparigrah* (**non-accumulation**): Non-accumulation of material assets is called *aparigrah*.

Aparigrah is a higher state of *asteya*. In the practice of *aparigrah*, we not only get rid of the desire to steal, we also give up our own unnecessary possessions. The lust to accumulate one material asset after another is *parigrah;* and the opposite is *aparigrah*. Common interpretations include living with the minimal needs of life and not receiving any gifts. Gifts bring obligation and feed the desire to accumulate more material things. Also, gifts and possessions make our happiness conditional, by tying it to those objects. The concept of *needs* versus *wants* is used to give up all the unnecessary stuff. On one hand, being self-reliant is recommended; constantly giving into our *wants* develops bad habits, making us greedy and eventually resulting in an unhappy life. Narrowness of mind as mentioned in *asteya* is the cause of wealth accumulation. Other elements in addition to narrowness of mind, such as power, ego, don't allow a person to practice *aparigrah*. The practice of *aparigrah* invariably translates into a simple life. Simplicity is defined as an internal state, and its external manifestation varies. Yoga literature has quite some variation around the scope of *aparigrah*. The general recommendation is to focus on expanding our consciousness and to possess only enough to take care of our essential needs.

5. ***Brahamcharya* (sense control):** Restraint of all the senses is called *brahamcharya*

Brahamcharya means moderation in feeding our senses. The concept of habit suggests that whatever the senses get, they want more of it. The key point here is to be always vigilant about what we feed our senses. It is important not to suppress desires and feelings, but the intent is to get rid of the desire to feed the senses by wisdom. The topic of *brahamcharya* has quite a few different interpretations in yoga literature and is discussed in detail. The most common interpretation is to practice celibacy in order to restraint sexual desire. In this interpretation or hypothesis, a spiritual aspirant aims to control breath, *pran* (the life force), mind, and the vital fluid on the path to self-realization. Complete control over any one of these components provides control over the others as well. On the other hand, a conscious effort to control all four simultaneously is considered the fastest way. Giving into sexual desire is considered a definite way not to progress spiritually. For our purposes, let's put aside the spiritual aspect to keep it simpler. The restraint of senses is important for stronger will power and improved concentration, which are foundational for good decision-making and critical thinking.

Niyam, the precepts, include *shauch* (cleansing), *santosh* (contentment), *tapasya* (strict self-discipline), *swadhyay* (self-study), and *ishwarpranidhan* (dedication to God). These concepts need to be practiced regularly in support of the self-restraining principles of *Yam*.

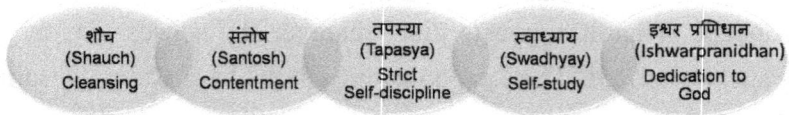

Figure 7: *Niyam* – The precepts for regular practice

1. ***Shauch* (cleansing):** Cleanliness of body and thoughts is called *shauch*.

The practice of *shauch* includes cleansing of body by proper bathing, yoga techniques, proper food, and so on. Cleansing of thoughts is done by constantly being vigilant of our thoughts. The guidance in yoga literature is to regularly practice being an *outsider* (observer without attachment) to analyze our own thoughts. The practice of *shauch* is supposed to prepare the "land" where the "plant" of concentration will grow.

2. ***Santosh* (contentment):** Staying content irrespective of circumstances and the fruits of our action is called *santosh*.

The concept of *santosh* is centred on satiation. The practice of being content all the time results in a peaceful and concentrated mind. The happiness produced by contentment is superior to the happiness produced by fulfillment of pleasurable desires. *Santosh* supports all five principles of *yam* and is the anchor to control desires. This should not be misinterpreted as a way to escape from our responsibilities. The goal here is to tame our desires and to calm the mind. A calm mind with fewer desires would suggest devoting time to more important activities. In yoga, the highest or "right" activity is meditation, which is defined as performing certain activity on our body to explore spiritual truths.

3. ***Tapasya* (strict self-discipline):** Regularly providing challenges to the body and mind in a disciplined way is called *tapasya*.

In yoga philosophy, *sanskaar* (the habits/impressions from prior actions) are deep-rooted. Bad *sanskaar* can be overcome only with the greater, positive strength which is acquired by *tapasya*. This includes conditioning of the body and mind with the proper kinds and amounts of diet, bodily training, and so on. The practice of *tapasya* gets rid of physical and mental laziness resulting in strong will power and a healthy body. This strength is the foundation to fulfill both spiritual and material aspirations. A life focused on convenience is bound to invite laziness and make us weaker. Without this self-disciplining practice based on consciously designed activities, it is also very easy to have inflated aspirations and the illusion of being knowledgeable.

4. *Swadhyay* (**self-study**): Reading and analysis of good literature is called *swadhyay*

Swadhyay includes introspection, acquiring knowledge, and conducting analysis. It is intended to enable continuous growth of mind. It increases the knowledge about the world, enhances analytical capability, and improves memory and our decision-making ability. In spiritual context, it also includes repeating the Scriptures. In the beginning, a yoga practitioner gets engaged in argumentative mental analysis to reach a decision/viewpoint on spiritual claims. Once he or she reaches a conclusion, the further effort in *swadhyay* focuses on intensifying that decisiveness.

5. *Ishwarpranidhan* (**dedication to God**): Dedicating the fruits of all our actions to God is called *ishwarpranidhan*.

This *niyam* suggests not taking any credit or any blame for the results of our actions, but dedicating all the results to God. This practice is intended to develop devotion and to keep a check on the ego identified with the body. *Ishwarpranidhan* is essentially a spiritual principle and one has to interpret it based on his or her viewpoint on spirituality. Most religions use this principle in the form of faith and beliefs.

A note on adoption and personalization of example guiding principles

It is important to note that practice of these principles is primarily an *internal effort*. Our behavior in the external world is only a reflection of our assimilation and internal practice of these principles. These guiding principles are not necessarily easy to adopt though. The adoption of these principles is not binary – yes, I adopted them or, no, I didn't. Based on our strength, wisdom, and ego, we adopt these principles to varying degree. In yoga, it might take multiple lifetimes to perfect ourselves. Scriptures suggest that actively expressing adoption of the arduous *yam-niyam* principles make us wiser and stronger to help us in our spiritual as well as worldly endeavors. As I mentioned previously, any convincing of our inability to adopt these principles should be considered an act of *maya*, the ignorance or illusion.

The *yam-niyam* value system is originally meant to be used at a *personal level* for *spiritual growth*. With their history and origin in spirituality, these principles have taken different forms in different cultures. Using this value system as an initial hypothesis and evaluating how different cultures have built traditions, would be an interesting endeavor in the field of social science. Typically, these traditions eventually become biases. In the previously introduced three-dimensional framework for analyzing people and societies, this bias due to traditions is perhaps the most prominent one.

The *yam-niyam* principles are an example in the *my*Life Framework. These principles also support both the foundational concepts of viewpoint on life – *balance* and *happiness* (mentioned in introspection chapter). One can experiment with these principles and use the appropriate language to personalize them. If these principles don't resonate with some of us, we have an option to develop our own guiding principles. Considering these principles as an example, you have the choice of developing your own guiding principles from scratch or using these as a starting point.

In the *my*Life Framework, the guiding principles are the anchor thoughts that drive our day-to-day behavior and, thus, need to be firm at every given point in time. Guiding principles are not supposed to be some idealistic thoughts that we simply appreciate. We rely on these principles to constantly make decisions to utilize the unknown amount of time left in our own life. These decisions shape our work buckets and the goals within each work bucket. So essentially, these guiding principles are the root of our achievements in life and dictate how we live life, day in and day out.

CHAPTER FOUR

The Work Buckets – An Example

The work buckets are a logical group of tasks that consume our time and mental energy. Considering humans as a single, inseparable entity, these work buckets are interdependent and need to be balanced continuously. Collectively, the work buckets should cover every aspect of an individual with no overlap among them; an overlap is a sign of cluttered thinking.

The primary viewpoint on work buckets definition needs to be of *balance* as opposed to *prioritization*. Prioritization is obviously critical for execution's sake, but taking a prioritization viewpoint has a danger of continuously deferring action on certain work buckets, due to less important things becoming urgent in one's day-to-day routine. Therefore, it is important to define a minimum amount of effort in each work bucket in order to qualify it to be on the list. The concept of primary identity, the central theme of a person's life can also be used for prioritization in crucial times. The *my*Life Framework highlights the importance of the primary identity by showing the corresponding work bucket in the center, as the polestar of all our work.

Just like the guiding principles and any other component of the framework, the work buckets can be changed anytime. They do need to be clearly identified and firm at any given point in time though. The work buckets are pretty broad and typically don't need to change often; it is a good idea to revisit the guiding principles and the work buckets once a year or so. The work buckets do have their own principles. For example, if *health* is a work bucket, a related principle could be, "eat only at scheduled times." It is important to keep the overall guiding principles separate from the work bucket principles. Ignoring the big picture, too many times people focus on a work bucket and dwell on its related principles rather than the foundational guiding principles, causing them to stay imbalanced and unhappy.

Overview of example work buckets

The work buckets I provide here are only examples to illustrate the *my*Life Framework and are a generic version of my own. You can use none, one, more than one or all these work buckets. I don't claim to be an expert in all these areas. In fact, it is mathematically impossible to learn everything about all the work buckets. To develop a viewpoint on work buckets, I have focused on the applicability of knowledge when synthesizing the essential information on these topics. Therefore, the thoughts here are the essentials of each work bucket as I understand them, but you should evaluate the information here, and throughout the book for its quality and relevance to your life.

The example work buckets in no order of importance are spirituality, relationships, health, finance, learning, social contribution, and desire management. Figure 8 shows the example in graphic form.

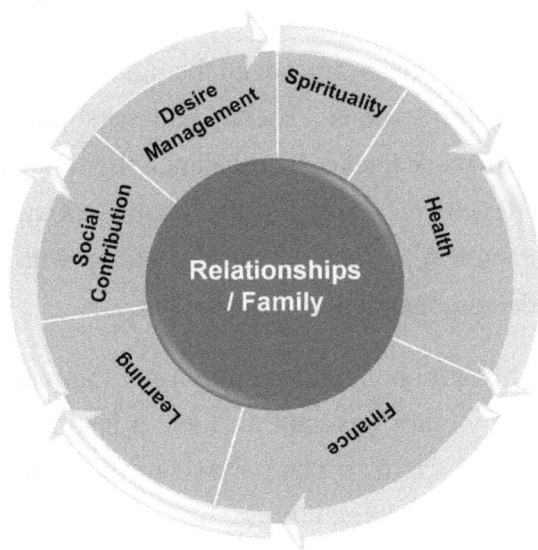

Figure 8: The example work buckets

Spirituality: Almost all of us are affected by religion or spirituality to some extent. People spend time on this work bucket in the form of improving their understanding of beliefs, practicing rituals, meditating to explore spiritual truths, and probably many more ways. The purpose of this work bucket is to capture the time and mental energy we spend on spiritual or religious activities.

I've used my understanding of yoga and spirituality as a key input to illustrate the *my*Life Framework. The content in this section of the book serves as an introduction to spirituality based on yoga theory. A good understanding of this section should give you a better context to all other parts of the book.

Relationships: Humans are social beings; we interact with people in our professional, social, and personal lives. The purpose of this work bucket is to balance the time and mental energy we devote to managing the people around us. This bucket is intended to include family, along with the other people inside and outside our personal lives.

Health: A healthy body is an important prerequisite to a quality life. If we are fortunate to have a healthy body, it is our duty to take care of it. The purpose of this work bucket is to strive for a healthy longevity.

Finance: Being financially self-reliant allows room for a person to aspire for higher human needs. Money is perhaps the next common denominator after time, as it can be exchanged for most of the things in society. The purpose of this work bucket is to manage the investment of our own life dedicated to earning money.

Learning: Proper education should teach us how to live a good life. Learning needs to improve our understanding of the world around us as well as our own being. The role we play in the world is decided by our understanding of the world. The purpose of this work bucket is to manage our effort to improve our understanding – of self and the world around us.

Social contribution: Since we take things from the world all the time, I believe it is our responsibility to give back *our share*. An individual can't be happy if the society around him or her is a failing one. Considering oneself as part of the world broadens our consciousness and contributes to our overall happiness. The purpose of this work bucket is to do our share in improving the world around us.

Desire management: If we consider the goal of life is to be happy all the time, then all the activities we do should be based on having fun. This is the *catch-all* work bucket that includes the activities we do for fun and the activities not fitting into other work buckets. The purpose of this bucket is to control the time we spend on *fillers* or *sponges* (things that waste time or suck it up but are unnecessary/undesirable) versus the things we really enjoy doing (that is, proactively planned, productive work).

Since all of us are unique to certain extent, the work buckets I've listed here are not meant to be the same for everyone.

The key takeaway here is to balance our activity in the given 24 hours of the day as well as the finite, unknown amount of time left in our lives. You can use the generic work buckets identified here as a starting point to develop your own work buckets.

The following pages provide an overview of the example work buckets. This overview is meant to illustrate the depth and breadth of the viewpoint needed on a work bucket. As I summarize my thoughts on very different topics, I'm sure to leave out more things than I cover in these pages. *Although you might find certain useful thoughts in these viewpoints, my goal in the following pages is to describe the myLife Framework.*

I've included yoga and spirituality in almost all of my analysis on life, but this does not mean that you must do the same. Although I have a yoga mindset, the *my*Life Framework is completely independent of the yoga philosophy. You should use my analysis only as a starting point to build the details around your own work buckets.

SPIRITUALITY

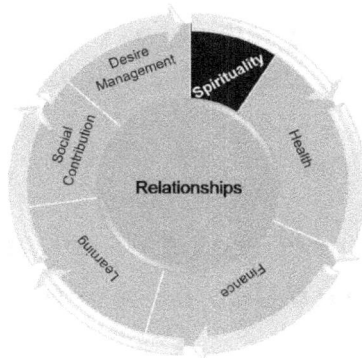

This work bucket captures the *time* and the *mental energy* we devote to religious or spiritual activities. The activities can range from improving understanding of our beliefs, practicing rituals, meditating to explore spiritual truths, or anything else you think of as spiritual or religious. If you don't consider spirituality as an element to be balanced in the *my*Life Framework you can skip this section without impacting the framework's utility.

A plethora of literature exists on spirituality, yoga, and religion. My goal here is not to add one more piece to serve the lust of mind for aimless analysis or to confirm or confront any religious beliefs. The thoughts here are simply a summary of my analysis on spirituality. The topic of spirituality is too vast for anyone to grasp everything across all religions. The content I've written here is based on what little I've understood from my experience and the analysis of the literature I have investigated. I invite you to evaluate my analysis, as well as the sources of my information. Three primary sources of my information on yoga and spirituality are the teachings of *Swami Vivekanand, Paramhans Yoganand,* and *Saint Kabir.*

The structure of all religions – Beliefs, rituals, and a value system

A common understanding in any field of study starts with a standard definition of the key terms that explain the concepts in that field. The words have been especially misinterpreted in the field of spirituality, so let's agree on the terms *spirituality, religion* and *yoga* for analysis in this chapter. For our purposes, *spirituality* is the field of study related to the existence of God and the individual soul or spirit within all living beings. God is defined as the super-conscious, the all-intelligent supreme soul, *the finest form of energy* (Additional explanation in later part of this section). The term *religion* refers to a specific path to explore the field of spirituality or the truths about God. Yoga claims to be the science of spirituality – the most scientific way to explore the spiritual truths. The word "yoga" literally means "union," signifying the union of an individual soul with God. The word "scientific" in this context refers to the ability for anyone to reach a common outcome by using a specific method.

With this understanding of spirituality, religion, and yoga, I looked at some of the religions (the paths to explore spiritual truths) and noticed a common structure across them. The common structure of all religions is that they all contain the three components of beliefs, rituals, and a value system.

- **Beliefs** are certain basic thoughts that a religion asks its followers to believe through faith, and typically without any proof. Proof is the outcome of any scientific experiment that can be experienced by all human beings using a prescribed method. As an example, we can't see the radio waves transmitted from a radio station to the radio sets in our homes. However, using the proper scientific knowledge, tools and methods, all of us can validate the existence of radio waves. Religious beliefs lack this universal experience. Our history is full of conflicts due to religions, or paths, trying to force their beliefs on each other without the ability to provide universal proof.

- **Rituals** are the practices or traditional activities of a particular path, like going to church, temple, synagogue or mosque, and following a prescribed set of behaviors.

- **A Value system** is a set of foundational principles (or the guiding principles, as I call them in this book) that drive the core thinking process for a religion's followers (For examples, the 10 commandments of Christianity or *yam-niyam* of yoga).

Collectively, a value system, beliefs and rituals seem to define the *way of life* recommended by any and every religion.

Yoga has a fourth component that is missing from most religions: a certain *meditation technique* that a yoga practitioner *applies on the body* to explore spiritual truths. In yoga hypothesis, the human body has a unique spiritual structure that can be leveraged to experience spiritual truths using certain techniques. In yoga practice, these techniques are the core element or, primary focus of the yogic way of life. These techniques focus a little bit on the physical body but primarily focus on controlling the mind and the breath.

If we look at the history, the founders of all religions and some of their followers claim that they have directly experienced certain truths beyond what our senses can capture from the physical world. This direct personal experience typically fades away with time, and religions are primarily left with the three components mentioned above – beliefs, rituals, and a value system. I'd like to believe that all the people who had personal experiences of God, spirit or anything beyond the senses practiced some kind of techniques on their body and mind. Practicing these techniques for personal experience is a lot harder than practicing rituals. A lifestyle based on value system along with rituals and beliefs, does provide the satisfaction of a purposeful life for the followers of a religion. For the leaders in society; the religion also becomes a basis of power and a way to control the masses.

Although there are significant differences in beliefs and rituals, the value systems across religions seem to have a great level of commonality. They align pretty well with *yam-niyam* principles of yoga as well. However, it is impossible to reach agreement on the beliefs and rituals across religions, which continue to be the cause of wars even today.

Two short stories provide a good analogy to illustrate the concept of *spirituality* and *religions*. In the first story, which you may already have heard, a few blind men came to know that an elephant was in the neighborhood. They thought that even though they couldn't see the elephant, they could feel it. As each one of them touched a different part of the elephant, he got a different impression of it. The blind man who touched the elephant's leg thought it was like a pillar, but the one who touched an ear compared it to a fan, while the one who touched the trunk thought the elephant was like a pipe, and so on. Each of them insisted that he was right and the others were wrong. The story could end in two ways. First, these blind men could keep fighting. Or second, some passersby could help these blind men resolve their conflict by telling them "the truth." This represents how spirituality, like the elephant felt to the blind men, is different things to different people.

In the second story, which you may also have heard, a frog falls into a well. As he meets other frogs in the well, he suggests the existence of the world outside that well. The other frogs, having not seen the outside world, argue that the first frog is wrong. This story could also end in two different ways – one positive and other negative. In the positive ending, the frogs of the well could become aware of the outside world, while in the negative ending, the frogs just keep fighting.

Both stories apply to most of us as we consider religion: Typically, we also live in our "wells" of religion, and make no effort to know anything outside of that well.

The structure of all religions – Applied to the yoga path

I use the same four-component structure of **beliefs, rituals, a value system,** and **a meditation technique** to provide an introduction to yoga as I understand it.

To understand yoga theory, I call *beliefs* – the "spiritual hypothesis." By definition, a hypothesis can be confirmed or denied after proper investigation.

I propose that *rituals* should be completely ignored on the journey to test the spiritual hypothesis. Certain rules of behavior can be defined by a yoga practitioner in everyday life, but these rules need to be identified or created only by an individual, – the yoga practitioner testing the spiritual hypothesis. Any form of organizational effort to influence the masses should be viewed as rituals and can be discarded.

Therefore, for the purpose of our description of yoga no rituals exist.

The *yam-niyam* introduced as the example guiding principles is *the value system* of the yoga path.

A *meditation technique* on the body is unique to the practitioner trying to explore spiritual truths. Indian history provides numerous examples of saints, "self-realized" people – the ones who were able to have direct experience with God, spirit or experiences beyond the senses. The spiritual hypothesis suggests that all these saints used a particular technique on the body to explore spiritual truths and taught the technique to their followers. Their followings eventually became specific religions and usually lost the techniques because beliefs, rituals and value systems were much easier to teach, understand, and practice. Thus, an individual who wants to explore the spiritual truths needs to learn a meditation technique, from an *appropriate* source.

The spiritual hypothesis, spiritual goal of life and the yoga claim

The spiritual hypothesis based on yoga theory suggests the existence of God and a soul in all living beings. As mentioned previously, God is defined as the super conscious, the all-intelligent supreme soul, the finest form of energy. This finest or most subtle form of energy is manifested as the whole universe, with lessening degrees of subtleness or increasing degrees of grossness. The literature explains the concept of God in different ways; this definition is provided to align with yoga theory and the spiritual hypothesis. The piece of God, in its pure form, within each living being is the individual soul. Except for the soul, everything else in living beings is the manifestation of the finest form of energy at different levels of grossness, and *keeps changing*. For example, the physical body is a grosser manifestation of the same energy than the human emotions or the decision-making intellect.

As part of the drama of creation, the mind (*mann* or *manas* in Hindi) attaches itself to the senses and the other grosser forms in the world around us. The soul, on the other hand, ever pure, never touched by creation, wants to merge into the all-intelligent supreme soul – God. This struggle of the soul to merge with God and the effort of mind to stay attached with the senses and the creation is an ongoing one. This struggle is called the war of *mahabharat* in the holy book *Geeta*. An individual constantly identifies oneself either with the soul or with mind to take different sides in this war.

The goal of all living beings in this spiritual hypothesis is to merge with God. Merging with God is called different things in different religions: the *moksh*, salvation, self-realization, etc. A soul may take many lifetimes and different forms of life during this journey, but all souls eventually merge with God, with the completion of *one cycle of creation*. In philosophy, one descending and one ascending cycle of the four *yugas* form one year of God or one cycle of creation. A *yug* or *yuga* is specific period of time, during which most souls have a specific set of characteristics; higher a *yug*, closer most souls are to God. In the first half of a God year, the descending cycle of *yugas*, living beings become increasingly ignorant of the existence of finer forces and the existence of God. In the second half of a God year, the ascending cycle of *yugas*, the living beings gain the intelligence of the finer forces and eventually all merge into the supreme soul, God. In this flow of souls away from God and merging back into God, some individual souls are ahead while others lag behind. At every point in this cycle of creation, certain self-realized souls – the souls that are permanently merged in God, live on the Earth. Their purpose is to guide the souls striving to merge with God. Philosophers disagree on the amount of time it takes to complete one cycle of creation and on where humanity in general is, in the current cycle of creation: some say, humanity is still on the descending part of the cycle, while others suggest we've come out of the darkest times and have recently begun the ascending cycle.

The spiritual hypothesis suggests the existence of a soul within our bodies. Based on this hypothesis, the goal of each human is to make a conscious effort to experience, realize, or come face-to-face with his or her soul. From our very childhood, we focus on the external world; yoga suggests turning our focus inside to realize our true selves as souls, and provides certain techniques to help us do so. These yoga techniques pull the energy from the grosser forms and divert it to the finer spiritual dimensions. Only human beings have this ability to apply yoga techniques to realize one's soul. This is the reason that a human life is considered very special and different from other living beings. Only a human body houses a certain spiritual structure that can be leveraged to expedite the spiritual evolution. All other living beings, although have a soul, they don't have a conscious control of their spiritual evolution, and must follow natural progression.

All the activities we perform in this life cause certain results and leave impressions for the future. The actions are called *karma,* and the impressions left for the future are called *sanskaar.* (*karma* is sometimes also defined to include both action and its consequence). The *sanskaar* from this life and the previous ones form habits, which we sometimes collectively call the basic nature of a person. Since these habits are often stronger than a person's will power to counter them, many people believe in fate. Yoga teaches that an individual has full control over his destiny and that we should live life as guided by the soul, countering the past bad *karma,* the negative *sanskaar,* and the corresponding negative habits.

Yoga suggests that we are a soul, a piece of God himself, who created the whole universe. We are capable to do anything and everything by identifying ourselves with God. If we are not able to finish the journey of merging with God in this lifetime, the law of *karma* dictates that we'll continue the soul journey in the next life, picking it up right where we left off in the previous life.

Ways to achieve spiritual goals

Scriptures provide different ways to achieve this spiritual objective of souls merging with God. In his commentary on *Patanajali's Yoga-Sutras* (Chapter II, *Sutra* 25), *Swami Vivekanand* provides a good summary of different ways to reach the same spiritual goal:

"Each soul is potentially [undemonstrated or unmanifested] *divine. The goal is to manifest this divinity within, by controlling nature, external and internal. Do this either by work, or worship or psychic control, or philosophy – by one,*

or more, or all of these – and be free. This is the whole of religion. Doctrines, or dogmas, or rituals, or books, or temples, or forms, are but secondary details."

As suggested by *Swami Vivekanand* above, the four ways to achieve one's spiritual objectives are: work, worship, psychic control, and philosophy. Other yoga teachers classify the paths to spiritual progress differently. For example, one common way to reclassify these four paths is the path of knowledge, the path of devotion, and the path of action. Essentially, they all seem to cut the same cake in different shapes and sizes. Another way to look at these paths is to compare them with climbers scaling a mountain. When they are near the base, the climbers cannot imagine the existence of any other paths but their own, as they cannot see them. After reaching a certain height, they start learning about the different paths. When they arrive at the top, from the apex of the mountain they can see all the different paths that led to the top. In the same way, the four paths mentioned above may seem different in the beginning but eventually provide the same results.

Two great scriptures that provide deeper and additional context around *Swami Vivekanand's* four paths, as well as to the overall philosophy of yoga are: The holy book *Geeta* and *Maharishi Patanjali's Yoga Sutras,* – the yoga aphorisms. There might be other scriptures, but these are ones that I analyzed a little bit. One probably needs a lifetime to grasp these scriptures fully, but I'm sharing some thoughts about the four spiritual paths based on what I have understood so far from these two scriptures.

Work: This is also called the path of *karma* in literature. An activity qualifies as work only if it is done without an expectation of the outcome. Along with the activity being performed without attachment and expectation, all the fruits need to be dedicated to God. Not everything we do in life is qualified as *work* in this definition. Meditation is considered the highest form of work or activity. As mentioned previously, meditation is defined as the technique performed by an individual on his or her body for spiritual evolution.

Worship: This path of devotion is the most commonly used by religions across the world. Devotion is the manifestation of our emotions directed towards God. If devotion doesn't come to a spiritual aspirant naturally, yoga teachers suggest earning devotion by practicing meditation techniques.

Psychic control: This path focuses on controlling one's mind and emotions to build strong will power. It also relies on the yoga techniques of meditation, as well as a *yam-niyam* based way of life.

Philosophy: This path relies on complete detachment and complete rationality to see things in their true form. In order to see anything in its true form, one should have already overcome any attachment to the body and the ego. This detachment is accomplished by pursuing the same way of life and practices as are done in other paths.

The thoughts about each of the four paths are not mutually exclusive and, in fact, a yoga practitioner uses elements from all the paths to live a spiritual life. An individual focuses more on a particular dimension than the other dimensions based on his or her natural inclination. This *focus* results in the concept of yoga paths. To a large extent, the concept of "yoga paths" seems to be nothing more than words to explain the same central point: some of us are naturally action-oriented, others are devotional, and still others are more analytical. To me, these paths simply signify the dominance of an aspect within us.

Eventually, every path is supposed to help us reach the common goal of *stillness* or *quietness*. The saints suggest that, as soon as a practitioner can perfectly calm his or her mind, body and emotions, the spiritual experiences begin to manifest naturally by the law of cause and effect.

In the same way as several different words are given to these paths, a lot of "types" of yoga are mentioned in the literature. They also simply signify the dominance of a particular human aspect in an individual's effort to achieve the same spiritual objective. The path of *rajyog* or *raja yoga* is the most accepted and most comprehensively documented. It is structured in eight sequential steps to provide a maturity path for a practitioner. Numerous books describe the eight steps of *rajyog* in great detail, but here's an effort to summarize the commonly accepted view of *rajyog*.

The first and second steps of *rajyog* are *yam* and *niyam*, as I described them earlier. This is the value system to drive a spiritual way of life. It is intended to produce self-control and calmness of mind. The third step of *Asana* is intended to develop the ability to comfortably sit in a particular posture for a long time in order to practice meditation techniques. Any motion in the body needs to be controlled as it is a distraction for meditation by bringing the attention to the body. The fourth step *pranayam,* is considered the best tool in a yoga practitioner's toolkit for spiritual progress. *Yogis* say, our consciousness is tied to the energy in our body and *pranayam* aims to control and channel this energy. With the practice of various *pranayams*, yoga practitioners gain control over mind and physical aspects of their bodies, like heartbeat, and pulse along with preparing the spiritual structure inside our spine. *Pratyahar*, the fifth step, signifies the disconnection of our senses from the outside world at will. The practice of *pranayam* enables the practice of *pratyahar*. The sixth step, *dharna,* is one-pointed concentration, which is to be focused on God. This step is possible only after the mind is interiorized and disconnected from the senses. In the seventh step, *dhyan*, a practitioner prolongs the concentration and continuously gains knowledge from the object of focus, which is supposed to be God. So a yogi gains the vastness of God via feeling or intuition. Typically, this is the step we call meditation. And in the eighth step, *samadhi*, the practitioner dissociates his or her mind from external object of concentration and internally reflects or merges with only its meaning. A yogi merges his individual consciousness with the cosmic consciousness. Multiple stages of Samadhi are discussed in literature, when a yogi is able to discriminate and merge with specific internal states of mind.

In essence, the yoga *way of life* includes *spiritual attitude*, *balanced activity* based on a person's role in the world, *a meditation technique* and *devotion*. This way of life is supposed to *still* our body, mind and emotions, so that we can realize the existence of finer forces that our physical senses cannot capture, while effectively playing our worldly role.

- The spiritual attitude is based on *yam-niyam* as the value system or guiding principles of life. Another way to represent spiritual attitude is the goal of staying in the four identified states of mind – friendship, sympathy, being happy and indifference. It suggests being a friend of all, being sympathetic or merciful towards the suffering of others, being happy for the people when they are happy and being indifferent when people or life presents negativity. A yoga practitioner constantly watches out for these four states of his or her mind to keep it calm.

- Balanced activity is about proactively planning the investment of time across personally defined work buckets. Gradually, the yoga practitioner spends more and more time in meditation due to detachment from the external world.

- A meditation technique practiced regularly and with intensity is aimed to prepare our body and mind to experience spiritual truths. A proper technique detoxifies the body and improves a practitioner's control over the life force energy – the fine form of energy that sustains our body. A yoga practitioner tries to find a self-realized teacher to learn this technique. In addition to spiritual benefits, the practice of this technique is invariably expected to improve concentration, calm the mind, and improve will power, along with providing physical health benefits.

- Devotion is an integral part of the spiritual quest. The scriptures suggest that meditation techniques can take a yogi to the door of God, but one needs devotion to go through it. The practitioner is warned not to become superstitious in the name of devotion. *Swami Vivekanand* suggests that being a non-believer is better than being superstitious. A yogi earns devotion by the sincere practice of meditation techniques and his personal experiences.

A lot of guidance on spirituality is very mystical, so how do we figure out whether the efforts we are making are in the right direction? *Swami Vivekanand* suggests that "strength" be the primary test in determining whether to accept or reject anything spiritual, accepting anything that makes us strong and discarding it if it makes us weak in any way. In addition to the primary test of strength, his literature also provides comprehensive criteria to believe in spiritual claims.

So what?

I developed this viewpoint on spirituality after talking to many people, reviewing many sources of spiritual information and with some practice on the body. The big question for me was whether to believe in this spiritual hypothesis and test it or to discard it without proper investigation. The logical thing was to investigate it before accepting or discarding it altogether. The decision to investigate is, of course, not a simple one because it changes our whole way of life: It involves analyzing our own thoughts, controlling ego, and taming the wild horses of sense pleasures. I needed a few positive examples, along with a good rationale, to make such a huge change in my life.

As I evaluated the pros and cons of accepting and rejecting this spiritual hypothesis, I found myself in an interesting negotiation game within. The benefits of a good value system and the proven physical and concentration benefits of yoga were very clear. The claims of many spiritual people in support of this hypothesis made me think: If I don't pursue this, what if I wasted all the years of my life on meaningless things? On the other hand, it was simply not easy to change my regular way of life. The final decision from this initial analysis was to balance multiple things in life and to test the spirituality hypothesis on my own. This automatically led to the *my*Life Framework presented earlier.

Spirituality became one of the work buckets while making sure it helps achieving the goals in other work buckets as well. Conveniently, the framework is flexible enough to allow an increase or decrease in the effort in spirituality or any other work bucket in the future as needed. Additionally, considering spirituality as a work bucket in the *my*Life Framework provided me a way to dance with the mystery of life, with the thought that I might figure it all out one day or maybe not.

This section on spirituality is longer than the sections on the other work buckets of the *my*Life Framework. I felt it was necessary to provide this much context to make the framework more meaningful for people who consider spirituality an important aspect of their life. Even if you are not one of those people, I hope this content provides an improved perspective for the guiding principles.

RELATIONSHIPS

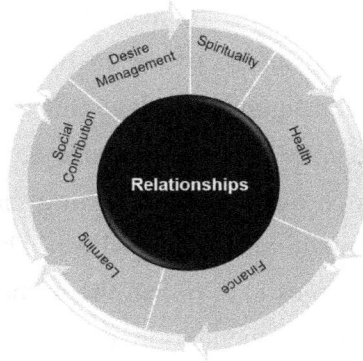

We are social beings, and having relationships with the people around us are a fact of life. The reasons for these relationships and their quality vary significantly. We love some people to death, and some we may hate passionately. In fact, for many of us, our relationships (specifically our family) are the primary focus of our lives. Considering the importance of family to most of us, I initially named this work bucket *family*, but I later changed it to the broader term "relationships."

Right or wrong, we devote a significant amount of time and mental energy in managing our relationships. Considering the management of relationships as a work bucket, I hope the thoughts presented here will help you manage the investment of time while improving your relationships.

Ego and image management

Relationship management starts deep within us and very early in life. We create an image of *me* in our minds, attach our egos to it and work diligently to place this image in the hearts and minds of everyone around us. Once we have placed the image *me*, we attach our egos to anything that is "mine" and start placing the image *mine* everywhere. The next step after placing all these images is to polish them, maintain them, and protect them. Every commendation about any of these *images* makes us proud and happy, and every assault on any of them makes us sad and angry, and prompts us to protect them. Overall, this image management is a lot of work!

In yoga theory, the ego (called *ahankaar*) is the last thing a practitioner gives up before making significant strides on the path of spirituality. So, the need for ego satisfaction and recognition is a very deep one. I'm not suggesting it is right or wrong to serve the need for recognition and appreciation; I'm only highlighting the significance of this *image/ego management* element, the amount of effort it takes and its impact on our relationships.

Purpose of relationships

Getting recognition is not the only reason we have relationships. We *need* people in our day-to-day lives for all sorts of reasons. In fact, this *need* factor is, perhaps, the reason for most of our relationships. Going beyond the *need*, we like spending time with our well wishers. We choose to spend time with people who have similar value systems and similar interests as ours. We don't have the complete freedom to choose relationships all the time though, as we inherit a lot of family-based relationships by birth. So, we have an option to choose relationships in most cases, but not all the time.

Using the personally identified work buckets provides a boundary for our needs. Putting a boundary around our *needs* also provides the rationale for having most of our relationships. For example, the *finance* work bucket suggests our need to get along with people in the work environment. The *learning* work bucket suggests getting along with people who provide guidance in our lives. An effective use of work buckets can probably cover all the reasons to have any kind of relationship. Besides the reasons that support our work buckets, ego satisfaction and emotional needs are perhaps the only additional reasons to have relationships.

I don't mean to suggest that we should have relationships only for some selfish or superficial reasons, nor am I recommending reducing the number of relationships we have by using the rationale of work buckets. In fact, good relationships are central to a meaningful and fulfilling life. The primary thought here is to be aware of the reasons for our relationships.

The concept of value exchange, loss of value, and human consideration

Virtually all human relationships are based on the concept of value exchange. Probably the exceptions come only when we include spirituality into the value exchange equation. The value is decided by the person on the receiving end. For example, a person might prefer a personal item from childhood memory over a very expensive gift, so he or she might *value* an old picture over a diamond watch. The word *value* does not have any meaning in itself unless the receiving person gives it a meaning in his or her own mind. In relationships, the value equally takes the form of material things, such as money from an employer, as well as intangible things, like ego satisfaction and emotional fulfillment.

Along with the value exchange principle, I've applied the concept of *energy efficiency* to human relationships. The concept of energy efficiency, which I learned from my physics class in high school, says, "*A perfect energy-efficient machine that would convert all input energy into useful output energy is an impossible dream. Converting one form of energy into another form always involves a loss of usable energy."* In the same way, expecting the "input value" provided by one person in a relationship to be equal to the "output value" received by another person seems to be an impossible dream.

The concept of value exchange is not comparable to a trade of things in a business deal; still it does apply to the depths of human relationships. A mother's love is considered supreme among all forms of human love. However, imagine how a mother's behavior would change, if the child kept disrespecting and hurting the mother for years? Even in a mother/child relationship the value exchange needs to be balanced for a quality relationship. Along with this concept of value exchange, we always need to remember the significance of being considerate as human beings. The golden rule of "treat others as you want to be treated" summarizes being considerate pretty well.

People often complain about not getting enough back from their relationships. Obviously, that's a sign of imbalance in the value exchange equation, for which there can be many reasons. The concept of value exchange suggests that we be rational and considerate for our relationships to be successful. In addition to being rational and considerate, the recognition of inherent loss of some value in the exchange process suggests that we give more into relationships and expect a little less. Typically, the opposite happens. People seek to get more from relationships without investing enough. Part of the reason for this is that many people have an inflated sense of self-worth and for the value they offer, while underestimating the value of what they receive from others.

All of us are expected to take care of ourselves, but people often take this "me first" attitude to an extreme and focus only on extracting value out of relationships, becoming selfish. An effective value-exchange relationship does require some level of maturity on both sides of the equation. Without making this psychological analysis very complex, the point is: a properly balanced value exchange is critical to all effective relationships in the long run.

Expecting change vs. acknowledgement, acceptance and appreciation for differences

When something goes badly and a situation is tough, typically the first thing we do is blame someone for it. After blaming them, we expect them to change. We expect the change not only in their behavior but also in their foundational way of thinking! This blame game and expectation of change is, perhaps, not the wisest approach. First of all, the focus needs to be elevated to the overall situation at hand. Many times, no one is to be blamed; it is the external circumstances and not a person that is responsible for a poor outcome. Even if a person is responsible, it might not be because of his or her intent. The poor result might be because of his or her ignorance, lack of capability, poor communication, or anything else beyond his or her control. So, more often than not, the responsible factor is something other than the *intent*.

Even if the intent of a person is in question, he or she might be simply taking care of self. We need to differentiate between the person's genuine need to take care of self from being just plain selfish. Even if a person behaves only for self-interest and doesn't provide value to us, I prefer to think of him as unwise, rather than selfish. This judgment, criticism, and "issuing character certificates" to people in our minds, is a slippery slope for our own growth and a poison for our relationships.

Indeed, when people are really responsible for bad situations or outcomes, it is mostly because of their lack of capability, or they are simply being unwise. Humans are inherently imperfect and expecting (sometimes even demanding) perfection is unfair and unrealistic. Taking the focus beyond the people and acknowledging their weaknesses and ignorance help us be more effective in specific situations, as well as in the overall relationship management. This approach also helps us practice the concepts of being rational and considerate, which are the keys to good relationships. In fact, *Saint Kabir* suggests keeping a critic close by to constantly purify and improve us. We learn more from the people who are different from us, so instead of disliking them we need to appreciate the value they provide.

Expecting a positive change in others is usually a big expectation. The crafty and strong forces of *maya,* or nature, are hard for all of us to overcome in order to make a positive change. Furthermore, the power of old habits makes this change even harder. Unsolicited advice and pushing people to change only brings resentment. If we decide to help someone make a necessary change, we can probably do only two things. One is to provide them an example of the change in our own behavior, and two is to try creating the right environment for the change. Keeping a check on our change expectations and being comfortable with a diverse group of people may or may not bring the desired result in specific situations, but it is definitely critical for our own peace of mind, which is the basis of right decision-making.

Yoga principles and relationships

Although the practice of yoga principles is designed for an individual's spiritual progress, they are very applicable to getting along with people as well. The principle of being truthful builds credibility, and the principle of non-violence takes away jealousy and makes us a well-wisher of all. Additionally, the principles of non-stealing and non-accumulation focus on self-reliance. The yoga concepts suggest that human behavior is always unreliable until it is anchored in God or divinity. The purpose of relationships with imperfect human beings, whose ordinary love is rooted in selfish desires, is to let spiritual aspirants practice the concept of unconditional love. It is our nature to seek love and connection with God and with his reflection in other human beings. The concept of individualism and being self-centered goes against these yoga-based ideas. I understand, these thoughts may sound too idealistic or saintly to some of us. Thus, one has to make up his or her own mind whether to weave these ideas into their personal life.

Human beings are complex and their interaction in relationships is not simple. Applying the thoughts presented here is not necessarily going to make us friends with all people. After all, the other people in the relationship equation might have a completely different mindset. Relationships involving family issues, traditions and religion are very tricky, but I do believe that applying these concepts can definitely improve our relationships while maintaining our peace of mind.

I've often thought of this farmer's story as an appropriate summary of my viewpoint on relationships. A certain farmer used to win the award for "best crop" in the region every year. When a journalist asked him for the secret behind his repeated victories, the farmer responded simply "I use the best seed available in the market and I share my seed with my neighboring field owners as well. Sharing my high-quality seeds with neighbors is probably the only unique thing I do. If they use poor-quality seed, then the weeds will grow in their fields and will come to my field in the wind and spoil the crop." In the same way, as external environment is of utmost importance, it is only wise to surround ourselves with the right people and help them in any and every appropriate way.

HEALTH

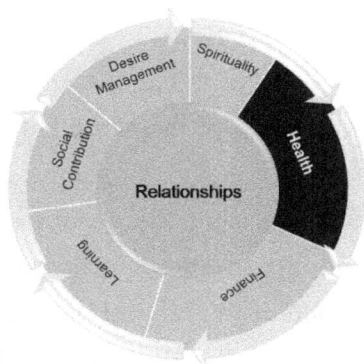

I once read a statement posted on the wall of a natural therapy center in India, which translates as, *"Being ill is a sign of your ignorance, stupidity, and laziness."* It made me burst into laughter from the blunt way it was written, but after a while I thought, "Yes, it is true that we are responsible for taking care of our body. Can we really call ourselves mature if we don't take care of it?" Later, I read a statistic in a health book that confirmed the same thought. It mentioned that 85% of the health problems that doctors dealt with could be either prevented or solved by patients themselves. This required people to comply with the natural rules of staying healthy, like eating the right food and getting adequate rest and exercise.

The challenge of staying healthy has only increased in recent years. A study by Harvard Medical and Law School in 2005 suggested that half of personal bankruptcies in America are triggered by healthcare costs. So, health is not only a matter of quality of life at personal level, it is a real challenge to govern societies across the globe. Popular culture is driving a lifestyle with very little physical activity, no discipline in eating habits (eat anytime, all the time, fast food, stale food, etc.), and the quality of food is worsening due to the use of fertilizers and food processing. As a similar lifestyle spreads across the world along with growing populations, healthcare could very well be one of the biggest menaces we face in the future, if we are not already there. The point is to acknowledge some of these macro factors and make a conscious decision to take charge of our health.

A traditional Indian saying is that health is the first of the seven blessings of a good human life. (The others are enough wealth, a good wife, an obedient son, a residence in your own country, a share in the social power structure, and contentment.) I believe most of us would agree that health is a work bucket in the *my*Life Framework. However, while all of us recognize the importance of health, not all of us make an effort to stay healthy.

The purpose of this section is to provide an example viewpoint on health as a work bucket in the *my*Life Framework. My thoughts in this section are based on my understanding of yoga, acupressure, and food. This section is not intended to provide a complete health guide. Numerous health books exist to serve that purpose.

Understanding of the human body – It's complex!

A human body can be viewed as a complex living machine. This complex machine is essentially a series of integrated systems. Each system has a specific role that it performs in perfect cooperation with other systems to maintain the overall health of the body. The static view of our body or its systems is studied in anatomy. Specifically, these are skeletal, muscular, nervous, endocrine, cardiovascular (circulatory), respiratory, reproductive, integumentary (skin, hair, and nails), lymphatic and immune, and urinary (excretory) and digestive systems. Each of these systems is made up of organs that consist of tissues and tissues that are made up of cell. Cells are considered the most basic building block of our body.

This static view is complimented with physiology, which is the study of these systems in action. Physiology focuses on the dynamic chemical interaction at the microscopic level. The health of the body is dependent upon our genetic inheritance and how well we treat it. While genetic inheritance is out of our control, we do have control over how we treat it.

With this understanding of the human body from our high school biology class, what does it mean to be healthy? At the basic level, the cells need to be healthy and, as we go up in hierarchy, the organs need to be healthy and the body systems need to work properly. Then all the systems need to work together well; for example the skeletal system, the muscular system and the integumentary system, along with all their lower elements in the hierarchy – organs and cells – need to work together to provide us appropriate physical support and movement. As the body systems interact with each other, information needs to be transferred effectively through the levels of hierarchy and across the body systems.

Although we may not notice it from the outside, our body is mostly fluid. About two-thirds of our body is composed of water with many substances dissolved in it. Our body's cells and tissues are delicate and require certain chemical and physical equilibrium to function properly. Multiple systems work together to keep this balanced environment.

There is no way for all of us to grasp all the details of our body. Still, to maintain it properly, we need to have essential knowledge about it. At the very minimum, we need to recognize the complexity of our body. We need to acknowledge this fascinating miracle of our body as we use and misuse it every day.

Yoga perspective – Even more complex!

It is an amazing feature of our body, or us humans, to be self-curious. Scientists are studying the body in more detail every day. *Yogis* and the ancient *rishis* (saints or spiritual scientists) did the same. I've shared my understanding of their messages as the hypothesis in the spirituality work bucket section of this chapter.

In yoga perspective, just behind the physical structure of the body, an even subtler spiritual structure exists. The mental and feeling elements lie between the physical and spiritual levels in terms of subtleness. The finest form of energy, which is eventually responsible for a body's birth, well being, and death is channeled through the spiritual structure. Yoga suggests the superiority of mental (and feeling) aspects over body and the superiority of spiritual aspects over those mental aspects. The spiritual structure being so fine, it cannot be explored with the physical instruments of the external world. Saints suggest controlling the mind and will power to channelize the finer forms of energy through the spiritual structure. This is exactly the purpose of *pranayam*, which is more commonly interpreted as special breathing techniques to improve effectiveness of oxygen usage in the body. As a yogi's practice matures, his or her body physically changes to enable the spiritual progress by reorganization of the finer energies in the body. In support of physical health, yoga also suggests that an unhealthy body is an obstruction to spiritual experiments, and it is our divine responsibility to take good care of it.

Obviously, the documentation about yoga perspective is mostly obscure and not easily provable. I'm not sure how many formal organizations are doing a disciplined research on this topic to develop an authoritative view for the world. My point is to identify these claims about the existence of the finer forms of energy further than what we learn in our biology class. As we start merging the biological understanding of our body with this yoga perspective, the analysis to keep the body stronger for a longer time becomes even more complex!

What to do about this complexity?

With the complexity presented above, it is simply not possible for all of us to become experts in every aspect of our whole being. So, with the goal to take care of our health, how do we address this complexity of body? I think the first thing to do is to acknowledge this complexity and take responsibility for our health. We cannot rely only on doctors and become the subjects of their experiments for ongoing research. Unfortunately, more doctors simply fix certain breaks rather than providing holistic patient care. Even if they have the expertise and right intent to help, eventually we are responsible for our health.

The next logical step is to build the essential understanding about staying healthy. Now, what is the scope of this "essential understanding"? The scope vaguely lies somewhere between knowing everything written in yoga or biology books and mistreating the body. Every culture has certain norms to stay healthy. Without becoming biased towards or against them, we need to leverage the experience of our past generations. I don't think it is wise to simply ignore the experience and undocumented empirical data of our past generations.

With the goal to obtain essential understanding and leverage the experience of past generations, I have experimented with *yogasans*, *pranayam*, acupressure, food, and some general health rules to address the complexity of maintaining health. Diseases do not develop overnight. They are a result of breaching the rules of health and ignoring the body signals repeatedly. In the event of facing common health issues, I've successfully experimented with the natural ways of treatment from Indian tradition. I have found some of these methods in books and some from personal knowledge of people around me. While, it is true that the body is complex, but its maintenance can be simple. I believe that, by complying with natural health rules, it is very much possible to stay healthy and to avoid the doctors in 85% of the cases, as mentioned in the beginning of this section.

Food, yogasan, pranayam, and acupressure

It is not possible to go into great detail to explain food, *yogasan*, *pranayam*, and acupressure in this small section. Only a brief synopsis of these topics is provided here. Further exploration can be pursued independently.

Food is the primary source of energy for our body. The energy generated from food is the key to our cell-level health and a balanced chemical environment of various systems. Although a lot can be written about food, I'll mention two points of practical use. One is that *digesting* is more important than *what* we eat. If we are able to well-digest the food we eat, in all probability we are eating right. The other practical point is that typically our digestive system is overworked and fasting helps remedy that. The benefits of fasting go beyond simply resting the organs. *Yogis* suggest that most common diseases can be cured by judicious fasting.

Yogasan or *asana* is the third step of *rajyog*, which provides exercise to every part of the body including the internal organs. At the most basic level, *yogasan* physically tenses and relaxes all the body parts. Regular practice of it makes the body parts strong yet flexible. It helps remove toxins and enables the smooth flow of all the body fluids, which in turn helps the physical and chemical equilibrium of our body. The practice of *yogasan* is much more comprehensive and much different than regular physical exercises, which focus primarily on muscular and skeletal systems. *Yogasan* practice releases all the blocked energy and removes local tensions to prepare our body for an effective *pranayam* practice, which is the next step in yoga practice.

Pranayam is controlling and channeling the life force energy. It is done with the combined effort of the breath, the mind, and will power. Because it involves breathing in a disciplined way, *pranayams* are often referred to as breathing exercises. Although the description around the control of life force energy may be hard to prove and understand, *pranayam* practice increases the amount and effectiveness of oxygen in our body. The body uses this extra oxygen for detoxification. The workload on the heart and other body systems decreases with higher purity of the blood. The practice of *pranayams* is perhaps the most effective way to clean the body and keep it healthy at the cell level.

Acupressure is the art of treating diseases by applying pressure on specific points in our body. The pressure is applied typically by a thumb on the points where the pain exists. Like yoga, the principle of acupressure is also related to channeling the finer energy throughout the body. Although its origins and rationale might be argued, I've seen its effectiveness on myself and the people around me. The approach of applying thumb pressure on our palms and the soles in areas corresponding to where we feel pain is so simple that anyone can easily learn and practice it.

One may argue about these concepts and theories, but the benefits of *yogasan, pranayam,* and acupressure have stood the test of time. By using some of the techniques from these topics or other similarly proven ways, I believe we can stay away from most ailments. If you have no background on these topics, learning and adopting these might sound a bit daunting. In fact, anyone can learn the essentials of *yogasan, pranayam,* and acupressure within two to three months. Then it is a matter of daily practice of about 30-45 minutes a day to stay healthy.

FINANCE

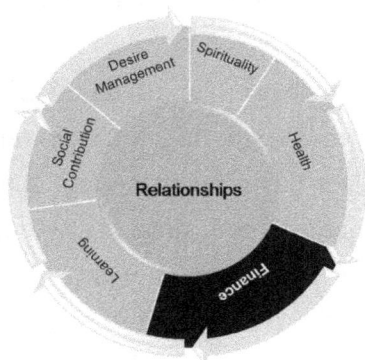

Making money is the work bucket that consumes a significant amount of our precious time, typically more than we want to devote to it. Of course, money is important. It can be exchanged for a lot of things in life and most importantly for our precious time. Somewhere deep inside us, we believe a lot of money will cure all the issues in life and make us happy. Yes, one cannot be self-reliant without having enough money to meet basic needs. A lot of people take money's value to the extreme and consider it synonymous with a successful life. It is hard for many of us to differentiate between financial success and a successful life.

What's our viewpoint on money –
Its place in our lives?

I've presented finance as one of the work buckets in the *my*Life Framework. Considering finances only as one of the buckets, at the most basic level money is only a tool. This tool should help one live a desired lifestyle and it deserves a finite investment of our time and effort. In the same way, all of us need to have our own definition of being wealthy or financially healthy. Without this basic viewpoint, we can't evaluate our success.

In addition to a basic definition, all of us need to have some essential thoughts, our viewpoint on money. These essential thoughts form the foundational attitude that impacts our everyday behavior and drive actions to earn such wealth.

Is money good or bad? Many of us think money is the root of all evil. Some of us, particularly those among us who believe strongly in capitalism, may say that it is the root of all good. We may think that we need to sell our souls, be unethical, or live a stressful life to make money. We may think that rich people have made money via only wrong means and still we want a lot of it. I remember having similar thoughts when I was in high school dealing with fellow wealthy classmates. But now, I believe we need to have a positive attitude toward money. It is a useful tool to accomplish many things in life and we don't need to sell our souls to earn it. We also need to understand and evaluate where our beliefs on money come from.

In the current trend of consumerism, I've come across many people whose only way to be happy is by *spending money*. Consuming stuff and spending money is sort of their religious ritual. Asked to think of something fun that doesn't involve spending money, they come up blank. I know quite a few people who live this high-earning, high-spending lifestyle. They spend a lot of energy earning money, and they spend a lot of energy spending it. They watch television or interact with people who make them feel that the only way to be happy is to consume more things. This earning and spending cycle is simply not sustainable for most of us. We need to evaluate our personal situation and priorities to develop a viewpoint on money.

How much money is enough?

For spiritual people, guidance on "how much money" is very clear from many sources in Indian scripture. The principles of *asteya* (non-stealing) and *aparigrah* (non-accumulation) suggest a lifestyle focused on simplicity and enjoying the fruits of our hard work. Saint Kabir says, "God give me enough to take care of my family. Anyone who comes to my door also should not go empty handed."

Our needs vary depending upon our viewpoint on life, our external environment, and our attitude toward money. Ideally, all of us would want to have enough of it so that we don't have to think about how much we spend. In reality, we need to evaluate our personal situation to build a definition of being financially independent. To set our financial objectives, we need to know our own capabilities, the environment around us, and where we are starting from. The starting points of a 55-year-old illiterate person, a teenager middle-class boy, and a kid inheriting some fortune are completely different. Being financially self-reliant to take care of our needs is a prerequisite to being happy. At the same time, earning a lot of money is not enough to be happy.

To emphasize that we must be comfortable with what we possess, a traditional Indian saying goes, "Stretch your legs based on the size of your bed sheet." Another traditional Indian quote suggests poverty is the worst thing and the company of saints is the best thing that can happen to a person. So money is a very useful tool and we should make an honest effort to earn it. At the same time, money is not a cure for all the deeper issues inside us. We need to have a talk with ourselves to define a place for money in our life and then come up with specific financials goals to be achieved.

How to reach financial independence?

Once we have our definition of wealth and have identified realistic financial objectives, it is a matter of building a plan and executing it to achieve these objectives. One way is to align our true interests with the profession we choose. I can't imagine a scenario when a person's profession is aligned with passion and he or she retires financially poor. Of course, there's an element of practicality. One can't expect to be rich doing things that no one is willing to pay any money for.

Broadly, I see three paths to earning money. They are working as an employee for someone, running a business independently, or building wealth from investments. Depending upon our interests, capabilities, and the path we take, the scale and lifestyle varies significantly. In each of these cases, we need to manage the financial equation of money flowing in and flowing out with timing. Along with improving my professional skills, I've used the *yam-niyam* guiding principles of non-stealing and non-accumulation in this equation. These guiding principles essentially focus on self-reliance and ask us to define our needs versus wants. I have personally invested more of my mental energy and time on learning and personal development, rather than saving or spending money. For me, less mental energy spent thinking about saving or spending money helps me to stay detached and fight greed.

For most people, the current trend of globalization only adds to the financial uncertainty in coming years. Continuous learning to stay informed about the world around us, enhancing professional skills, and better planning for uncertain times is the need of the hour. A one-time career planning activity in college days to predict the rest of one's life seems to be a luxury of past generations. In today's fast-changing global work environment and with the overarching concept of acquiring debt to contribute to a capitalist economy, we need to be careful not to acquire more debt than we can afford. And considering the uncertainties of current times, we need to plan our savings accordingly as well.

Applying the cause and effect principle, a pragmatic plan to earn the right amount of money can be developed. Too many people focus on the constraints limiting their financial objectives and narrowing the viewpoint of life itself. I've noticed that many people who think big, in fact, only imagine big. They are too lazy or incapable to even develop a pragmatic plan to achieve their financial goals. If we are able to develop plans, we need to remember that the results are due to the actions; the plans are not enough. As in any other aspect of life, we need to have a foundational viewpoint on wealth, some specific goals, and actionable plans supported by an effective execution of those plans.

Just like we learn music from a musician, guidance from financial experts should be followed on this topic, and I'm definitely no financial expert. I'm sharing the thoughts I've acquired from my experience and my thoughts here are intended only to illustrate the financial viewpoint in the context of the *my*Life Framework.

LEARNING

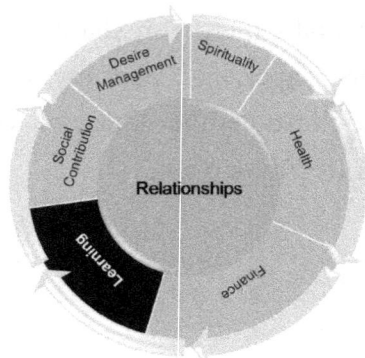

The first four buckets of spirituality, relationships, health, and finance are applicable to most of us, as we typically all devote a lot of time in those. I'm not very sure how many people really devote enough time in *learning*, to call it a work bucket in itself. Still, I believe we should and that's the reason *learning* is an example work bucket here.

The purpose of learning

As mentioned in the introspection chapter, I have three expectations from education or learning. They are:

1. It should provide us the professional skills to earn a living.
2. It should answer the question, "How do I live a good life?"

3. It should make us contributing members of society.

The first expectation is pretty straightforward. Depending on one's profession in life, a personalized professional development plan provides the scope of learning. The goal for this bucket is to make a mark professionally along with helping us earn a good living.

The second expectation about answering the "how to live" question is a complex one. Depending on a person or culture's basic viewpoint on life, the scope of learning would vary. The scope includes something similar to the basic thoughts provided in this book. The scope also includes the essential knowledge in the work buckets. For the example in this book, learning is expected to provide essential knowledge on yoga, spirituality, health, human psychology, relationships, personal financial management etc.

The third expectation on being an asset to society rather than a liability typically comes only when certain prerequisites are met. These prerequisites include meeting the basic needs in our hierarchy of needs. A good education first helps a person in meeting their basic needs and also provides the right mindset to be a socially responsible individual. People with the fortunate situation of having their basic needs met, obviously have more flexibility to choose a socially responsible role.

I can imagine a true high-quality life only for a learned person. Saints say, "Ignorance is the greatest sin." We cannot tackle challenges we don't know about. The only way to counter ignorance is to improve our understanding, of self and of the environment we live in. Only with a good understanding of the world around us we can play an effective role in it. The need for this improved understanding of the world has only increased with the globalization trend of current times.

Mental traps on the path of learning

Obviously, the kind of learning I'm talking about is not directly related to the degrees offered in the formal educational system. True learning provides the appropriate knowledge and inspiration as well as enables the continuous growth of mind. Learning focuses on knowledge relevant to improve our condition in life. Most people seem to lose interest in learning after completing their formal education. By definition, learning requires being interested in things we don't know about. However, many of us only spend time on the topics we know about and are comfortable with. In the name of learning, many people simply look for confirming data to validate their preconceived notions. Many of us focus on acquiring information for conversational pleasures or to serve our mental lust for analysis. Experience also works as a deterrent for creativity, innovation, and learning as a whole.

In the yoga context, the path of knowledge is considered superior to the paths of devotion or action. They say knowledge is power because, when a yogi gains true knowledge of self, he or she is no longer affected by *transient* nature all around. Yoga theory also suggests learning, or *swadhyay* as a regular practice. In spirituality, along with the body, "doubt" is considered one of the initial hurdles in spiritual progress. A disciplined learning effort helps eliminate these doubts by providing appropriate knowledge and inspiration.

I think knowledge itself is enough reward to justify the significance of learning, besides its practical use. Based on its significance in yoga literature, the suggestions from the great ones, and having seen its utility in personal life, I consider learning a work bucket in the *my*Life Framework.

SOCIAL CONTRIBUTION

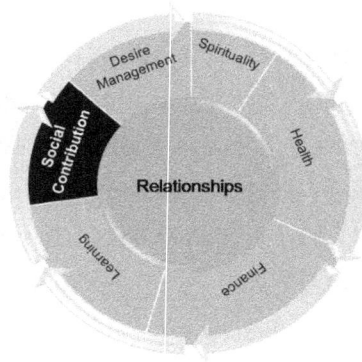

For our purposes, let's define social contribution as time we devote to activities that help improve the society we live in. These activities don't provide any direct tangible benefit to us, to *me,* or to anything or anyone we call *mine.* Just like learning, social contribution may be difficult for many people to consider as a work bucket. In fact, this one might be harder because someone else *seems* to get the benefits of the time we invest!

Why be socially responsible?

So why invest time in social responsibility activities? Reasons for people vary significantly, from material gains and emotional satisfaction to altruistic, from deep compassion to serving God. I'm sure there's a well-researched, long list of reasons for people to get involved in social service activities. I have a few reasons of my own for considering social contribution as a work bucket. If you don't think social contribution should be a work bucket for you, the *my*Life Framework is obviously flexible enough for you to ignore or replace it.

Without putting the reasons in any logical order, fairness comes to my mind as the first valid motivation for social contribution as a work bucket for me. We extract so much from the world we live in, it is a matter of fairness to put our share back in the system. If we don't contribute our share, the system will deteriorate and collapse with time. Simple logic suggests that if our external environment is not what we want it to be, sooner or later it will impact us at a personal level as well. The farmer's story of sharing the high-quality seed with neighboring field owners illustrates the same point. So, in fairness, it is simply our responsibility to do our share to improve our external environment. Also, it is better to do it without inflating our egos or considering ourselves better than the rest of the people around us.

The second reason for being socially responsible is a more fulfilling way of life. Once our basic needs are met, we have a choice of where to invest our time. Among all the options of focusing on family, making unlimited money, having fun, and a lot of others, making a positive contribution to society seems to be a good alternative. What we include in our definition of *basic needs,* of course, varies by individual and personal circumstances. Even when our basic needs are not met, there is some social role for all of us. I believe taking care of our social responsibilities will enhance our capability to take care of personal needs as well. To me, the scope and timing of contribution may vary by circumstances of an individual. But considering social responsibility an important aspect of one's life definitely makes it more complete and fulfilling.

The third reason is the expansion of consciousness. As it relates to the five *yam* principles of yoga, narrowness of our mind prompts us to be violent, to steal, and to accumulate material assets. As a small example, I noticed someone being jealous of a neighbor's garden, rather than enjoying the beautiful flowers and landscaping. The person's narrow consciousness didn't let her enjoy nature's beauty. Expansion of consciousness is very helpful for spiritual aspirants due to its multi-dimensional benefits. This is perhaps one of the reasons many religions suggest getting involved in social work.

The example of role models is another reason for me to consider social contribution an important aspect of life. All the people I respect have contributed to society at large without keeping any selfish motives as the center of their lives. Although I believe in the independence of my own thinking process, I also feel comfortable simply following in their footsteps.

Thus, some personal rationales along with the examples of role models are more than enough reasons for me to consider social contribution as a work bucket.

No need to take on the burdens of the world

Sometimes we believe that taking care of society is only the government's job. A little bit of analysis suggests that nobody really has enough control or ability to drive the world, the nations, or even the smaller regions within a country. Sometimes even the intent to serve society at large is missing.

At the world level, globalization and unprecedented scarcity of natural resources seem to be the central themes of our times. With the world so tied to the concept of *growth* (not progress), we are heading for a crisis if we are not already there. With the growing pace of exploiting natural resources, the consumerism-focused way of life is simply not sustainable. While no single government controls these macro trends, all of us have our share of impact on it.

Maybe there is a profound, divine purpose behind the global changes and commotion, or maybe not. With an improved understanding of what's happening around us, there's a role for all of us to make a positive impact on the societies we live in. This need is at all levels – from local to national to global. However, it is important to remember that no single individual can bear the burden of the world; we need to think about doing only our share.

Obviously, one option is to ignore this social role completely. Another option is to improve our understanding of the world around us and then maybe take up an appropriate role for us. That's a personal decision. I've included social contribution as a work bucket for your consideration because of our inherent connectedness to nature and the people around us.

DESIRE MANAGEMENT

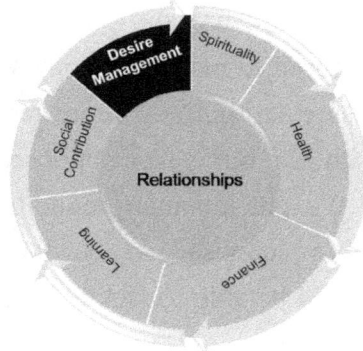

When I identified the initial list of work buckets, some activities that consumed my time did not fall in any of them. Life is supposed to be fun and I did not have a placeholder for the fun activities. So I created a bucket called "fun." Creating a bucket for the fun activities quickly related it to the concept of desire fulfillment in spirituality. The theory suggests that all human desires need to be fulfilled. The accumulation of pleasurable events generates desires for more of the same and their unfulfillment will bring pain eventually. Be it good or bad, end of the day, both types of desires are obstruction in the spiritual progress. To address this, we have two choices. The first one is to keep creating the new desires and to keep fulfilling them. The second option is to fulfill selected ones and simultaneously get rid of certain desires with wisdom. Thus, I renamed this work bucket from the lively name "fun" to a more generic name "desire management."

It is very easy for kids to be happy, but with age, the smile fades away. It takes too much effort for us to be happy and still we call ourselves mature and grown up. All the small things that are supposed to make us happy somehow become meaningless or less exciting. Yes, more responsibilities and pressures come with age, but we are supposed to be wiser and stronger as well. We put too many conditions on us to be happy, whereas it's supposed to be the opposite. With experience, we should be able to tackle the challenges of life without affecting our smile. This work bucket is a placeholder for the activities that support this goal of being peaceful and happy every day. It also gives an opportunity manage our viewpoint of life as collection of pleasurable events versus pursuing the goal of even-mindedness.

This bucket can be used to capture all the activities we *want* to do and that are not covered in other work buckets. This bucket can also be very helpful in managing things we do due to the pressures from our external environment versus the things we want to do independently.

Using this bucket along with others must provide a placeholder for every activity that takes our time. Activities not included in any of the work buckets need to be considered as *fillers* or *sponges* – meaningless, unenjoyable things that consume our precious time.

WORK BUCKET INTERDEPENDENCY

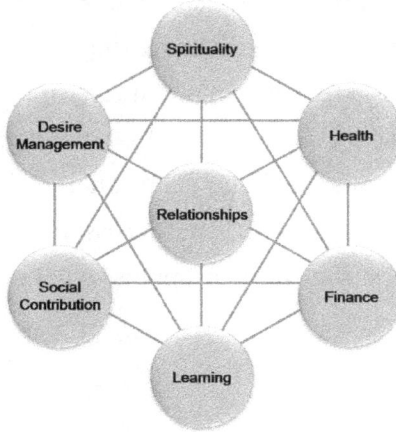

Figure 9: Work bucket interdependency

The work buckets I've mentioned here are only an example to demonstrate the application of the *my*Life Framework. The framework itself is a skeleton that needs to be filled by personalized work buckets depending upon the things important to an individual. The thoughts I've shared within each work bucket are meant to provide examples of viewpoints on each bucket and the associated level of detail. A lot of *rules* tend to come up when building the work buckets and these rules need to be differentiated from the overall guiding principles of the *my*Life Framework.

The work buckets, by definition, are supposed to be mutually exclusive. Collectively, they are supposed to capture every activity that consumes our time. This criterion of mutually exclusive and collectively exhaustive is a good test for the clarity of thinking. As humans are a single, inseparable entity, the work buckets are very much interconnected. The goals within a work bucket would typically have dependence on the factors in other work buckets. This inherent interdependence requires consideration of factors across the work buckets to establish goals and then develop plans to achieve these goals.

CHAPTER FIVE

Using the myLife Framework

Throughout the book, I've tried to focus on the applicability of concepts. But many of the concepts being so overwhelming, the focus might stay on philosophy rather than its implementation. As a clarification, note that execution is everything. Anything before execution is simply the preparation for it. In fact, *you should be able to connect every thought in this book to implementation in your own life*. If you are not able to do so, I suggest ignoring those thoughts, because there is danger of getting trapped by our ego and mind's lust for aimless analysis.

With the goal to prepare ourselves for implementation, the prior chapters of this book focused on the *description* of the *my*Life Framework. In this chapter, I share some thoughts on implementing the framework. My goal here is to provide you with enough guidance to start applying the *my*Life Framework (or some derivative of it) right away.

It's about change and change is not easy

Pretty much all of us think that we are wise and know most of the things we need to know. We usually have a pretty good *image* of ourselves. Still, most of us want to improve that image for ourselves and for the world around us. This improvement effort requires change. This need for change is primarily within us and much less for things around us.

For a number of reasons, change is not easy. People feel comfortable with the status quo and there needs to be some special reasons to move away from it. Human beings to a large extent are nothing more than what their habits are, as we are pretty much driven by the momentum of habits. Habits are deep rooted and hard to change. As we add the desires and ego dimensions to habits, change becomes even harder. The result is that typically people don't change; they simply become stronger in their essence with time. Real change has to come from within and requires a strong rationale and will power. In most cases, people either focus on superficial change or simply hope or *only have a vague desire for a positive change.*

Many people pass a lifetime with this vague desire to improve themselves. Saint Kabir says "hope and desires don't die, while the body dies life after life." We simply hope for change and generally make fragmented efforts to improve. The *my*Life Framework can be effectively used to transform this vague desire into concrete plans for execution. Obviously, the desire to change and plans to change are only the necessary initial steps before taking up actions to change.

Three enablers to change ourselves

I've observed three concepts in yoga literature with regard to driving deep change in a practitioner: The right external environment, the right knowledge, and sincere practice.

The right external environment keeps us in the company of people and situations that are conducive to the goal. In yoga, we have seeds of all sorts of desires inside us and only those desires will come up for which the environment is conducive.

The right knowledge provides true understanding; it dispels doubts and provides clarity of goals. This is accomplished with an honest introspection and constantly being vigilant regarding the things happening around us. Being vigilant requires staying detached and as unbiased as possible by observing things as an outsider.

Finally, the concept of *sincere practice* is used to develop positive habits and strength by repeated action. I heard the phrase "be sincere" in a yoga teacher's speech and since then I've always been able to appreciate the value of this phrase in execution. The use of the word "sincere" is very simple and can have a profound impact in our attempts to change our lives.

An approach to build good habits

Along with these three essential concepts, there's guidance for the maturity path or the sequence of steps to reach peaceful state of mind. Peace is considered a prerequisite for happiness and any spiritual experiences.

The first step in this approach is *resistance* or *staying away*. The suggestion in this step is to develop the strength to resist the temptation to get involved in negative situations or negative thoughts. Typically, we are tempted to fight bad habits or situations as soon as we face them. The recommendation is not to confront the negative external environment or internal thoughts or habits until we are strong enough to win.

The second step is *adherence*. The goal in this step is to develop the strength to adhere to positive thoughts and activities. These two initial steps on the path to mature in yoga practice or life in general – to stay away from negativity and focus on positives – are of utmost importance.

The first and second steps collectively build one's strength to practice the third step: *self-control*. In this step, yoga practitioners train their habits by conscious control of will power. *Pranayam* techniques are considered the key tool to build a strong will power. A yoga practitioner uses will power and *pranayam* to reach the goal of a peaceful state of mind. The peaceful mind enables a practitioner to make right decisions, and with the strong will-power (simultaneously built by the steps mentioned above), he or she smoothly progresses toward the spiritual (or material) goals.

In addition to this approach of staying away, adherence, self-control and *pranayam*, the eight steps of *rajyog* also provide insight for steps toward change. These eight steps of *rajyog* were introduced in the spirituality section of the work buckets chapter. Although multiple steps can be practiced simultaneously, the sequence of adoption has its own significance. As a recap, the eight steps of *rajyog* are *yam, niyam, asan, pranayam, pratyahar, dharna, dhyan,* and *samadhi.*

There are numerous ways to interpret and adopt yoga concepts. To drive change in a person's life, I've used the abovementioned three concepts, the maturity path, and the eight steps of *rajyog* to anchor my thought process. Once we have an anchor, it is relatively easy to identify the course of action for personal development.

Yoga-based thinking invariably leads to a lifestyle focused on simplicity and contentment. However, as people focus on getting away from material ambitions, many of them simply become lazy. The suggestion is to focus our efforts with fervor on spiritual progress, rather than focusing too much on unimportant material stuff. Many times, people use spirituality or other religious philosophies as an escape from the regular challenges of life. There's clear guidance that it is better to focus on enjoying the material world than being lazy. It is better to be a non-believer than to lose common sense and become superstitious.

An approach to adopt the *my*Life Framework

The overall approach of personalizing and implementing the *my*Life Framework can be summarized in three general steps:

1. Introspection – to what to change? (desired future state)
2. Tactical planning – how to change?
3. Execution – action to change!

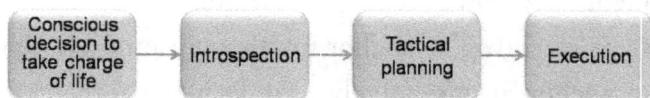

Figure 10: An approach to adopt the *my*Life Framework

After making the conscious decision to take charge of life, the **first step of introspection** is perhaps the most complex and most challenging for most of us. It is because we are trained to analyze only external objects. In addition to training, we have certain tools and techniques to evaluate the external world. Introspection requires the mind to analyze itself. It requires separating a part of us as an observer while the other part of us conducts everyday work as the object of analysis. This is not an easy task; it requires appropriate training and, more importantly, a lot of sincere practice.

The purpose of introspection is to build a *story of our life* and tell it to ourselves. Introspection requires that we evaluate our upbringing and the nature we've inherited from our parents. It includes questioning ourselves and identifying the central themes of our lives, those things that are most important to us. In relation to the *my*Life Framework, introspection identifies our guiding principles, builds a list of work buckets, and builds a viewpoint on life. Furthermore, it sets practical goals within each work bucket. These goals need to be directionally clear and could be vague in term of *end state* as some of these might be farther out on the time horizon.

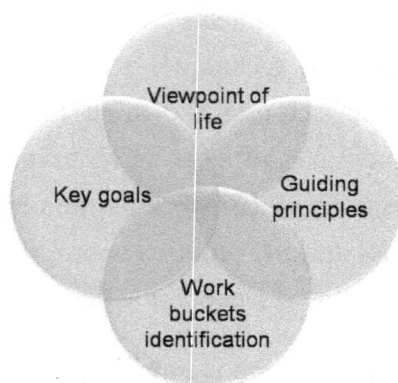

Figure 11: Outcomes of introspection

Introspection does require a minimum level of knowledge and some experience in life. Most of us seem to build the story of our life between 20 and 30 years of age. The age matters, but still the attitude to learn and act takes precedence over age. As I mentioned previously, without taking charge, our story of life is subconsciously built by the world around us. In this story, typically the definition of success includes power, fame, and wealth accumulation, as well as other elements respected in a particular culture. There is nothing wrong with this definition as long as it aligns with something deep inside us. As this is not our personalized definition, there is a danger of misalignment. If that happens, we are bound to get confused and eventually stay unhappy.

All of us build the story of our life differently, connecting our strengths, limitations and personal circumstances. It is only with this self-analysis that we consciously become aware of our capabilities and needs. The better we understand ourselves, the more likely it is that we'll choose the right role for us in life and be comfortable with our performance. If and when tough situations come along, this "self-consciousness" means that we are more likely to respond in consistent and effective ways. Along with the understanding of self, we also need to comfortably accept ourselves in our very *authentic* way. Too many times we want to become someone else. This introspection being a long journey is definitely not easy, especially with the appreciation for instant gratification all around us in popular culture.

The outcome of this introspection is the real test of our wisdom and maturity. It is important to watch out for the constraints we set around what's possible and what's not possible for us to achieve. In yoga theory, we are made in the image of God and we are capable of accomplishing everything. It is *maya* or illusion that tells us that we cannot achieve certain things.

Although introspection and learning continues throughout life, an initial viewpoint on life significantly reduces the turbulence of mind. The value of conducting this self-analysis sooner in life is pretty obvious to me, but it took me about seven years to convince a friend to make it a priority. If you are unable to firm up your views on the required outcomes of introspection, you may personalize the *my*Life Framework to define your initial viewpoint on life. Once we have a starting point, it is only a matter of refining it as we keep maturing in life.

The **second step of building tactical work plans** is a test of our critical-thinking ability. This is the step when we transform the conceptual ideas to real tasks to achieve our goals. In this step, we clarify, confirm, and put additional details on the direction we set for ourselves in step 1. Depending on how we set the direction in step 1, this could be a relatively simple task or a very involved one. From the example in this book, we have seven work buckets. Building seven detailed work plans could be mind-boggling. So, we might want to have details for some work buckets while only some high-level rules on others.

The idea here is to develop high-level tactical plans to accomplish goals within and across work buckets. These tactical plans need to identify the specific tasks in support of the work bucket goals while considering their interdependencies. The next step is to develop one execution plan of work for the foreseeable execution time horizon across all the work buckets. Depending on an individual's circumstances, this time horizon could be from a couple of months to a year or so.

Eventually, the *one execution plan of work* needs to capture the tasks to act upon, along with a personalized daily routine. Certain *anchor* activities are needed to adopt a daily routine.

Examples of these anchor activities are sleeping, waking up, or meditating at a fixed time of the day. I specifically want to highlight the significance of a daily routine or identification of tasks to act upon in the execution time frame. *Without this, all the prior glorious thinking could simply go waste.* Lastly, we do need a way to remember the outcomes of all the planning, *until the thoughts become second nature to us.* As an example, we may want to prepare a single, ready reference page with the key reminders from introspection, tasks to finish, and our personalized daily routine.

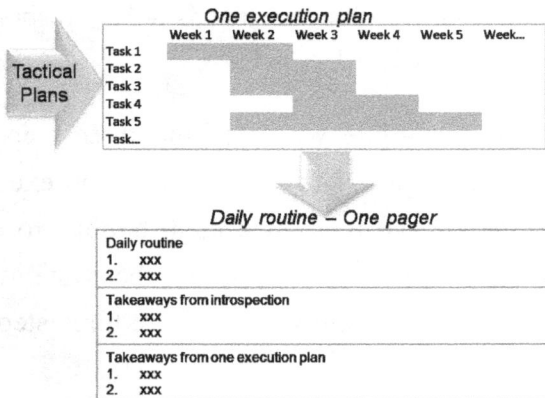

Figure 12: Outcomes of tactical planning

For some of us, this planning and organization comes naturally, while it might be an enormous challenge for others. Although it has taken me a great deal to explain the whole thinking process, practically, the tactical planning should be relatively simple if the basics are clear. A minimum level of analytical capability, which I believe all of us have, is the only requirement to plan the work.

The **third step of execution** is the real test of our strength and maturity. This is the *cause* we need to execute and the *effects* are bound to happen. The concept of focus is important for execution. Typically, we have too many distractions that take our minds to the past or the future. We need to separate the time to act from the planning phase. A personalized daily routine, tasks from one execution plan of work and clarity of goals help us stay focused on execution. Still, it is successful execution that is solely responsible for the outcomes we want.

It is of no use to argue which of the three steps is most important. Introspection, tactical planning, and execution are all essential and make their own contributions to achieving our definition of success. Just as all the systems need to function properly in a healthy body, these three steps need to work in sync.

Obviously, a lot more can be written about each of these steps; I've provided only the essential thoughts to get you started with the *my*Life Framework. I'd ask you to evaluate the time and mental energy you spend on the important items versus the *fillers* or *sponges*. If the answer is that you are spending too much of it on inappropriate things, I'm sure you can utilize many thoughts from the *my*Life Framework and guidance on its adoption.

Personalization and adoption of the *my*Life Framework

At the end of the day, the *my*Life Framework is only a skeleton with the components of guiding principles, time, work buckets, goals, tactical plans, an execution work plan, and a daily routine. It is important to note that an individual needs to personalize it for adoption. To some of us, it might seem like pretty common sense stuff, while others might find it overwhelming. I do believe it is a very powerful tool when used with discipline.

Some of the ideas I've mentioned, especially the yoga-related concepts, may not be easy for many of us to adopt or even to understand and assimilate fully. However, "easy" and "difficult" are relative terms that are based on our current habits and willingness to change. As a reminder from the two universal laws mentioned in the first chapter, perhaps the biggest trick *maya* or ignorance plays on us is to convince us of our inability to accomplish certain goals. While the *my*Life Framework can help us organize our lives better, it is our strength to execute that matters the most. Two armies of good and bad are fighting inside us, and the one we feed more is going to win.

CHAPTER SIX

Concluding Thoughts

We make detailed travel plans for any trip we take away from home. Why shouldn't we plan the journey of life? This book is intended to provide the essential thoughts to jumpstart the planning tasks of your own life. If someone has not identified the need for this planning, perhaps there's a need for change in perspective. All of us need to plan for a better future, unless we believe that life is only a matter of fate and that we are puppets in the hands of some supernatural power. I disagree with that view of fate and suggest that we are responsible for everything that happens to us.

The *my*Life Framework is universal, but needs personalization

Whether you agree or disagree with my viewpoint on any specific topic, the *my*Life framework needs to be personalized. The guiding principles and the work buckets in the book are intended to serve only as examples, so try not to get emotionally wrapped up on any single point I may have made here. As there are a lot of opinions on specific topics, it is important not to lose sight from the central theme of the book – the understanding of the *my*Life Framework. The framework is not something you can copy-and-paste from somewhere to your life. The framework should be viewed as a skeleton that needs to be populated by your personal state of affairs. It also should be viewed as a whole, like the human body, in which all the systems play their specific roles. As with the body, where it is unwise to argue whether the brain is more important than the heart, it is unwise to spend time worrying about which part of the Framework is the most important – it all works together as a whole.

I've used happiness as the universal goal and the balance of activities within a finite, unknown amount of time as the central concepts of the *my*Life Framework. The goal of happiness or some similar, positive feeling is truly universal. In the context of the *my*Life Framework, the concept of balance is also not contradictory to the concept of focus. In fact, we do need to focus on things important to us, and accordingly, the share of specific work buckets could increase or decrease. The concept of primary identity, the central work bucket in the framework, can also be used to help clarify priorities in life.

Although I've introduced the subjective concepts of happiness and balance as the foundation of the *my*Life Framework, you should have your own definition of a successful life, a definition that should come from honest introspection. In the absence of a sincere identification of what is important to us, our success will be defined by the world around us, and the definition of success provided by external factors is bound to be less than ideal for us. Once we know what successful life means to us, the concepts and analysis in this book can accelerate the viewpoints on important things for us and prepare us for execution. For some, the content in the book will help them identify their personal definitions of success.

I don't consider the *my*Life framework to be particularly innovative, although it is particularly *useful*. All of us subconsciously perform the activities mentioned in the framework, so I've discovered or simply identified what already exists. Additionally, I've put all the activities we do in life in a structure, to reduce randomness of our acts and have a better sense of direction in life. I do believe, though, that the *my*Life Framework is applicable to all of us.

Keeping our feet on the ground while evaluating the sophisticated philosophies

This small book has touched on a wide variety of topics, such as yoga and spirituality, health, psychology, relationships, finance, globalization and cultures, etc. Any effort to answer a comprehensive question like, "How do I live a good life?" has to consider a wide variety of subject areas. I segmented my thoughts in a few dimensions to answer this big question and to document the thoughts in this book. These dimensions include personal versus community issues, spiritual versus non-spiritual aspects, the history-present-future of individuals and societies, and the extraction of timeless values versus identification of contemporary values by maneuvering through a myriad of thoughts from a variety of sources. I encourage you to think about these dimensions as you personalize the information in this book. While we elevate the thinking in time, space and knowledge dimensions, we don't have to lose sight of the goal to utilize the information at personal level.

A note on contemporary trends and Indian culture

I see globalization as a very important trend of current times. As mentioned in the beginning of the book, globalization is not only about integration of economies, it is changing the value systems at a personal level and for societies as well. It is changing the power structure of societies, roles of government, and the way we live. It is *forcing change* in societies in very tricky ways, which is very uncomfortable for most people. In the context of this book, globalization presents new opportunities for us to change our lives and a lot of noise to answer the big question, "How do I live a good life?"

Immersing myself in the western world gave me a chance to understand it and to evaluate my own Indian culture better. As I understand, Indian culture is essentially based on the spirituality hypothesis that suggests taking a scientific attitude to figure out what is true, rather than focusing on what is my own or someone else's belief. The knowledge about the ability of every human being to explore spiritual concepts by using a prescribed method is India's special contribution to the world.

The *yam-niyam* value system is the foundational belief system that supports every spiritual path and serves as the common link across the sub-cultures of India. I invite the

Indian readers to evaluate this observation of *yam-niyam* as the connecting thread across Indian sub-cultures. I believe it is unwise to ignore the significance of *yam-niyam*, the essence of a culture that has been sustained for thousands of years.

You may have noticed my respect for the *Yam-Niyam* value system throughout the book. At a personal level, the *Yam-Niyam* value system provides a meaningful way of life, along with a promise of spiritual evolution. At the community level, it acknowledges the existence of the other paths to spiritual evolution and provides a basis for simultaneous peaceful existence. Indian heritage suggests combining spirituality and social service to lead a good life at the personal level but, today, the popular culture is pushing these values to the background, leaving a vacuum in place for a *way of life*. Currently, no clear set of principles dominate in our fast-changing world and, as many competing value systems try to fill the vacuum, only the time will tell what's sustainable and what's right.

Although I've made some comments about society at large in the book, I've done due diligence only to answer the personal questions. So my comments at the society level should be taken with a grain of salt. I've usually been comfortable making broader statements with the belief that if I can put the man together, I can probably put the world together.

A note on religion and spirituality

Religion plays a very important role in most people's lives. Religions have significant conflict when it comes to beliefs and rituals and, to only some extent, value systems. It is impossible to bring religions together based on factors that can't be proven, such as rituals or beliefs. Although I've introduced yoga as the core or basic science underneath all religions, I do not suggest that anyone change his or her religious path. A lot of people have benefited from every religion, so no religion is bad; only the poor interpretation of a religion is bad. I encourage you to enhance your understanding of your own religion and then compare it with the spiritual concepts presented in this book. I'm sure this will help you get a new perspective and renewed enthusiasm for pursuing your current religion.

Most of the time, science and religion are viewed as adversaries but I don't think we need to do that. Modern science is in a state of constant change to provide any conclusive viewpoint on many things and definitely on most spiritual claims. At the same time, a lot of conclusions from science are final. So, the understanding of modern science needs to be judiciously applied to develop our viewpoint on spirituality.

The last word

Because yoga is an ancient science and the basis of a lot of the analysis in this book, some readers may think that I recommend copying the old ways of life. That is not the intent at all. It is impossible to go back to past and I don't suggest that. My intent is to learn from history, extract some essentials on life from our heritage, and adopt them in our personal battle for a meaningful life.

For readers who don't believe in spirituality, I'd say that use the concept of the *my*Life Framework to improve your viewpoint of life and organize it better. Along with that, constructively critique the other concepts in the book and adopt them based on your natural inclination. For readers with spiritual bent of mind, I'd say exactly the same thing. Additionally, don't stop with the information I've presented in the book. Sincerely and quickly build your essential understanding on spirituality and get to execution sooner rather than later. Also, let's solicit help from the self-realized souls for our spiritual evolution.

The content of this book being an opinion on a very general topic of life, I'm sure you'll have thoughts in agreement and disagreement with it. The human mind being an imperfect instrument, I'm sure my analysis has flaws. Moreover, the message could be lost due to the limitations of language and my inappropriate usage of words. Please evaluate my basic hypotheses, assumptions, and analyses as you critique it and personalize it for your own benefit. Although I've learned from a variety of sources, my core thinking is influenced by yoga theory, so while evaluating my thoughts make sure you compensate for my biases towards yoga. I do hope this book helps some people to better organize their life and inspires them to improve it.

***

SHARE THE THOUGHTS

SHARE THE BOOK

***

GLOSSARY
AND
LIST OF HINDI/ SANSKRIT WORDS

This glossary and the list of Hindi and Sanskrit words are presented here to recap some of the key concepts discussed in the book. It is important to note that most of the words have a long history associated with them and are utilized with many different meanings. I'm explaining the terms and providing meaning of the words that mostly closely reflect their use in this book.

KEY TERMS & CONCEPTS USED IN THE BOOK

Introspection: Self analysis to answer oneself: How do I live a good a life? After the initial answer, introspection keeps tracks of one's *progress* in life.

Three dimensional framework/ analysis: Strength, wisdom and ego are three characteristics that can used to evaluate behavior of any human being. A certain nuance or derivative of these three characteristics can be utilized to evaluate communities as well as any circumstances.

Law of cause and effect: This law says, "If there's an action then there's always a corresponding result."

Law of Free will: This law says, "We always have freedom to make decisions."

myLife Framework: A skeleton of components that can be used to structure our lives. These components need to be personalized with our viewpoints with the right level of details. The components are guiding principles, time, work buckets, goals, tactical plans, one execution plan, daily routine and results.

Guiding Principles: A few foundational thoughts that drive our day to day behavior throughout life. This is one of the components of the myLife Framework.

Work Buckets: The categories of activities, where we spend our time and mental energy. Collectively these work categories must cover every aspect of our lives without any overlap. This is one of the components of the myLife Framework.

Yam: As sample guiding principles, a set of five self-restraint principles intended to keep a yoga practitioner focused on the path of spiritual development.

Niyam: As sample guiding principles, a set of five precepts, the directives that a spiritual aspirant practices regularly, i.e. invests time and mental energy regularly.

Yoga: Yoga is the way of life, for the people who practice it. Yoga is the science of spirituality – the most logical way to explore the spiritual concepts. Yoga literally means "union" signifying the union of an individual soul with God.

Spirituality: Spirituality is the field of study related to the existence of God and individual soul or spirit within all living beings. Another general way is, the field to understand life via understanding of finer forces that our physical senses can't capture and what modern science has not yet identified.

Religion: Religion is one specific path to explore the field of spirituality.

Saint: A self-realized person, someone who has found God. This meaning is more specific than many variations commonly used, from loosely any "good" or selfless person to the official designation as saint by a church.

Using the myLife Framework: Includes 3 structures: Three enablers of change, an approach to change habits based on yoga theory and an approach to utilize the myLife Framework

LIST OF HINDI & SANSKRIT WORDS USED IN THE BOOK

Ahankaar: Ego

Ahinsa: Non-violence

Aparigrah: Non-accumulation

Ashram: Hermitage

Asteya: Non-stealing

Brahamcharya: Sense control. The term has many explanations, mostly centered on celibacy.

Dharm or Dharma: The term is used with many different meanings: religion, purpose of life, role of an individual in life, duty, right thing to do or a specific meditation technique adopted by an individual is his or her body

Dharna: One-pointed concentration

Dhyan: A stage of self realization when practitioner gains the vastness of God via feeling or intuition

Geeta or **Gita:** The holy book of Hinduism that explains spirituality and the spiritual way of living. The explanation is at many levels from very technical/ scientific/ yoga focused to "how to live." Numerous interpreters have explained Geeta at different levels based on their understanding and based on the timely needs of society

Ishwarpranidhan : Dedication to God

Karma: Actions, sometimes also collectively the "cause and effect"

Mahabharat: Spiritually, the war within each human being. The struggle of soul to merge with God and the effort of mind to stay attached with the senses and the creation. Historically, a very famous war in India about 5000 years ago

Mann or **Manas:** The state of mind attached to senses. The term has many meanings mostly aligned with states of mind, typically to signify "heart" (that feels) or our "mind" that thinks

Maya: The ignorance or illusion

Moksh: Self-realization

Pran: Pran is the foundational form of energy that sustains life of all living beings. It is also defined as the life Force that sustains a human body. Maharishi Patanjali has suggested pran control as one of the enablers in spiritual progress, whereas later yogis have made a whole field of study on this concept.

Pranayam: Controlling and channeling of pran, the life force. Done with the help of specific breathing techniques

Pratyahar: Interiorization, the disconnection of our senses from the outside world

Rajyog or **Raja yoga:** The royal yoga, one of the paths in Hinduism to experience God, the eight-step path primarily credited to sage Patanjali

Rishi: Saint, sage or a spiritual scientist

Sanskaar: In the book used as the *impression* that is left after we have experienced the consequences of our actions or habits from our own prior action. It is used as a specific impression and also the sum total of all impressions. Literature has a quite a few other meanings.

Santosh: Contentment

Satya: Truthfulness

Shauch: Cleansing, of body and mind

Swadhyay: Self-study

Tapasya: Strict self-discipline

Yoga sutra: Yoga aphorism, in this book specifically referred to Sage Patanjali's yoga aphorisms

Yogasan: The practices of asanas (the third step of rajyog), to keep body healthy and to perfect a particular seating posture to practice meditation.

Yug or **Yuga:** A specific time period in God year with similar characteristics of all the souls.

ACKNOWLEDGMENTS

Neither the thoughts presented in this book nor its actual creation would have been possible without the help of numerous people. Although it is not possible to identify everyone whose contributions have resulted in specific thoughts mentioned in this book, I do want to acknowledge some specific individuals who either had significant influence on me or provided direct input for the book.

Gems of wisdom are scattered all over the place in my rich Indian heritage. Although I've learned specific lessons from a variety of sources, I owe my core thought process to Gurudev Pramhans Yoganand, Swami Vivekanand, and Saint Kabir. The proper understanding of conceptual ideas comes only with their adoption in everyday behavior. I owe all of my early subconscious training to my parents, who ensured good practice of the theoretical concepts to provide me with valuable lessons in life.

For the creation of this book, my wife, Bharti, deserves a special mention. She is the one who triggered the idea of documenting my essential thoughts on life for her and for our well wishers. In addition to making the book more presentable throughout the process, she is the one who has listened to me day in and day out as the thoughts in the book took their current shape. Along with her, I want to thank some of my friends and well wishers who have listened to my thoughts, have argued with me, and have provided their own take on the initial versions of this book. Thank you Meraj Mohammed, Chander Shekhar Chawla, Rahul Malhotra, Christine Sailer, Sartaj Singh, Nathan Ontrop and Pundarikaksha Baruah. I also want to thank Dawne Brooks for editing the manuscript, so that you can better focus on thoughts in the book and not my writing skills.

Finally, I want to thank you for reading this book. I know how hard it is to grasp many of the concepts mentioned in this book, as they question you at your deepest levels. If I was able to connect with you at some level, from the bottom of my heart I feel very honored and humbled.

Wishing you a successful life!

Sunil Sheoran
sunil@mylifeframework.com

ABOUT THE AUTHOR

Sunil Sheoran has been a yoga practitioner and researcher for more than 15 years. Considering himself a student for life, he focuses on identifying and connecting essential knowledge across various fields of study. Raised in India and immersed in western culture as a student and professional for more than 10 years has provided him a broad spectrum of experiences across cultures and walks of life. While he holds a master's degree, a patent in the corporate world, and is published in professional international journals, he doesn't consider professional accomplishments as a qualification for anyone to author a book on life. In fact, his thoughts in this book are perhaps a better introduction of him than his professional accomplishments.

For more information on him and this book, please visit www.mylifeframework.com.

www.ingramcontent.com/pod-product-compliance
Lightning Source LLC
Chambersburg PA
CBHW031513270326
41930CB00006B/397